Vertigo and Dizziness

Thomas Brandt • Marianne Dieterich
Michael Strupp

Vertigo and Dizziness

Common Complaints

Second Edition

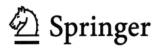 Springer

Thomas Brandt, MD, FRCP
Clinical Neurosciences and
Center for Vertigo & Balance Disorders
University of Munich
Munich
Germany

Michael Strupp, MD
Department of Neurology and
Center for Vertigo & Balance Disorders
University of Munich
Munich
Germany

Marianne Dieterich, MD
Department of Neurology and
Center for Vertigo & Balance Disorders
University of Munich
Munich
Germany

Additional material to this book can be downloaded from http://extras.springer.com

ISBN 978-1-4471-5925-4   ISBN 978-0-85729-591-0 (eBook)
DOI 10.1007/978-0-85729-591-0
Springer London Heidelberg New York Dordrecht

Preface to the Second Edition

The last 10 years following the first edition of our book have witnessed many new findings on epidemiology, diagnostics, pathophysiology, and – especially important – the course and therapy of various illnesses that have the main symptom of dizziness. It was therefore necessary to totally update the original edition, which had been conceived as a practical compendium of treatment strategies for patients with dizziness and balance disorders. Here we briefly highlight a few of the most important new developments.

Today valid epidemiological studies on the prevalence of various illnesses with the symptom of dizziness are available. The long-time course of benign paroxysmal positioning vertigo, vestibular neuritis, bilateral vestibulopathy, vestibular paroxysmia, Menière's disease, and phobic postural vertigo has now been investigated for over 10 years. Moreover, even physicians not specialized in this field are increasingly recognizing the clinical importance of vestibular migraine, bilateral vestibulopathy, vestibular paroxysmia, and the superior canal dehiscence syndrome. The diagnostic criteria have become more precise thanks to fruitful clinical studies. There is a wealth of new findings on the pathophysiology and central compensation of disorders of peripheral and central vestibular function, e.g., in the form of fMRI and PET evidence of plastic changes in cerebral activity. There are new data on higher spatial orientation disorders and on hippocampal atrophy in bilateral vestibulopathy as well as newly discovered vestibular structures and functions. We have covered these in the comprehensiveness needed for the private practice.

The following four findings are of special practical importance for therapy:

1. An important new therapeutic principle is the use of aminopyridine to successfully treat downbeat nystagmus, episodic ataxia type 2, and cerebellar gait disorders.
2. Corticosteroids significantly improve the recovery of peripheral labyrinthine function in patients with acute vestibular neuritis.
3. The most effective drug therapy for Menière's disease is evidently a high-dosage long-term therapy with betahistine.
4. Carbamazepine significantly reduces attacks in the long-term course of vestibular paroxysmia.

The personal experience of the authors has been gathered in the course of their engagement over many years in the multiregional Munich Dizziness Outpatient Unit. In 2009, the BMBF began funding this unit under a new name, the German Center for Vertigo and Balance Disorders (IFB). Its goal is to develop an international referral centre with an interdisciplinary outpatient unit, its own study centre, and a structured course of studies for foreign clinical scientists in the fields of otoneurology and neuro-ophthalmology.

In this second edition we would like to especially thank both medical and non-medical employees of the Dizziness Outpatient Unit, especially Ms. Sabine Esser and Ms. Ute Appendino for efficiently organizing the annual Munich seminar, "Vertigo," as well as the neuro-orthoptists Nicole Rettinger, Miriam Glaser, and Claudia Frenzel for carefully examining the patients, documenting each case, and compiling the videos. We would also like to express our appreciation to Sabine Esser for the graphic designs, Jenny Linn for her competent contributions to the imaging, and Erich Schneider for his development work on "bed-side" video-oculography. Our thanks also to Joanna Bolesworth of Springer Medicine UK for her pleasant, reliable, and extremely patient cooperation. Finally, we thank Judy Benson for her careful copyediting of the English edition of this book. The German second edition of the book "Vertigo – Leitsymptom Schwindel" by T. Brandt, M. Dieterich and M. Strupp was published by Springer – Verlag in 2012.

Munich, Germany   Thomas Brandt
                                                         Marianne Dieterich
                                                           Michael Strupp

Preface to the First Edition

There are three convincing arguments why it is important to learn about the management of vertigo:

- After headache, it is the second most common complaint of patients, not only in neurology and ENT departments.
- Most syndromes of vertigo can be correctly diagnosed only by means of a careful medical history and physical examination of the patient.
- The majority of these cases have a benign cause, take a favourable natural course, and respond positively to therapy.

Vertigo and dizziness are not disease entities, but rather unspecific syndromes consisting of various disorders with different causes. For this reason, our clinically oriented book is for physicians of different specialisations who treat patients with vertigo and for medical students. To make the book easy to use, we have provided an overview of the most important syndromes of vertigo and dizziness, each with elucidating clinical descriptions and illustrations.

A general chapter deals with how the vestibular system functions, its disorders, the pathophysiological mechanisms involved, diagnostic signs, history taking, examination procedures, laboratory diagnostics and principles of therapy. The most important clinical syndromes of vertigo are treated in individual chapters organised as follows: patient medical history, clinical aspects and natural course, pathophysiology and principles of therapy, pragmatic therapy, ineffective treatments, as well as differential diagnosis and clinical problems. We have put special emphasis on the various drug, physical, operative or psychotherapeutic treatments available. The book is based on the common experience that we have accumulated over many years working in a multi-regional referral centre for dizziness outpatients. Many parts of the text, tables and figures are updated versions of those in a considerably more detailed monograph on the clinical and scientific aspects of vertigo (Brandt T. *Vertigo: Its Multisensory Syndromes*, 2nd ed. Springer, London, 1999). The accompanying DVD presents typical case histories, results of examinations for the individual syndromes, physical examination techniques and laboratory diagnostics. The book is oriented to daily medical practice, and we hope that it will prove helpful by providing readily accessible information. The whole field of vertigo and dizziness, imbalance and eye movement disorders has been considered extremely difficult because of the variety of its manifestations and its resistance to compartmentalisation. We hope that we have succeeded in making these syndromes more understandable by using clear, anatomical categories and clinical classifications.

We would especially like to express our thanks to the neuroorthoptists Miriam Glaser, Cornelia Karch and Nicole Rettinger for compiling the videos. Our appreciation also to Ms Judy Benson for copyediting the text and to Dr. Steven Russell for carefully reading the manuscript. We also thank Ms Sabine Eßer for designing the graphics and Ms Melissa Morton and Eva Senior of Springer-Verlag London for cooperating on the production of this book in such a pleasant and efficient manner. The German edition of the book, *Vertigo-Leitsymptom Schwindel* by T. Brandt, M. Dieterich and M. Strupp, was published by Steinkopff-Verlag in 2004.

Contents

Chapter 1
Introductory Remarks

1.1 Physiological and Pathological Vertigo

Vertigo and dizziness are not unique disease entities. The two terms cover a number of multisensory and sensorimotor syndromes of various etiologies and pathogeneses. After headache, vertigo and dizziness are among the most frequent presenting symptoms, not only in neurology. The lifetime prevalence of rotatory and postural vertigo is around 30 % (Neuhauser 2007), and their annual incidence rises with increasing age (Davis and Moorjani 2003). Whether caused by physiological irritation (rotatory vertigo when riding on a merry-go-round, motion sickness, visual height intolerance) or a pathological lesion (e.g., unilateral labyrinthine failure or vestibular nuclei lesions), the resulting vertigo syndrome characteristically exhibits similar signs and symptoms despite the different pathomechanisms—dizziness/vertigo, nystagmus, a tendency to fall, and nausea or vomiting (Fig. 1.1). These disorders of perception (vertigo/dizziness), gaze stabilization (nystagmus), postural control (postural imbalance, falling tendency), and the vegetative system (nausea/vomiting) are related to the main functions of the vestibular system and can be associated with different sites in the brain (Fig. 1.2).

1.2 The Vestibular System

The most important functional structure of the vestibular system is the vestibulo-ocular reflex (VOR). The VOR has three major planes of action:

- Horizontal head rotation about the vertical z-axis (yaw)
- Head extension and flexion about the horizontal, binaural y-axis (pitch)
- Lateral head tilt about the horizontal line of sight, the x-axis (roll)

These three planes represent the three-dimensional (3-D) space in which the vestibular and ocular motor systems responsible for spatial orientation, perception of self-movement, stabilization of gaze, and postural control operate. The neuronal circuitry of

T. Brandt et al., *Vertigo and Dizziness*,
DOI 10.1007/978-0-85729-591-0_1, © Springer-Verlag London 2013

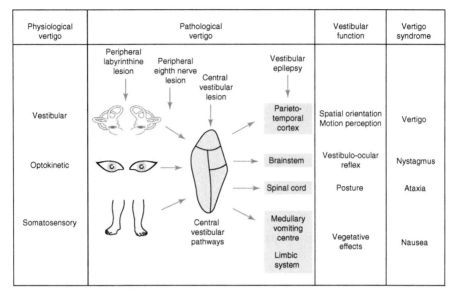

Physiological vertigo	Pathological vertigo			Vestibular function	Vertigo syndrome
	Peripheral labyrinthine lesion	Peripheral eighth nerve lesion	Central vestibular lesion		
			Vestibular epilepsy		
Vestibular			Parieto-temporal cortex	Spatial orientation Motion perception	Vertigo
Optokinetic			Brainstem	Vestibulo-ocular reflex	Nystagmus
			Spinal cord	Posture	Ataxia
Somatosensory		Central vestibular pathways	Medullary vomiting centre	Vegetative effects	Nausea
			Limbic system		

Fig. 1.1 Physiological vertigo (motion stimulation) and pathological vertigo (induced by lesions or stimuli) are characterized by similar signs and symptoms that derive from the functions of the multisensory vestibular system (reproduced with permission from Brandt and Daroff (1980))

the horizontal and vertical semicircular canals as well as of the otolith organs is based on a sensory convergence that takes place within the VOR (Fig. 1.2). The VOR connects a set of extraocular eye muscles that are aligned by their primary direction of pull with the same particular spatial plane of the horizontal, the anterior, or the posterior canal. The canals of both labyrinths form functional pairs in the horizontal and vertical working planes. In other words, the canals are stimulated and inhibited pairwise:

- The horizontal right and left pair
- The vertical anterior of one side along with the posterior canal of the opposite side and vice versa

  The vertical planes of pitch and roll are a result of the wiring connecting the two vertical canals that are diagonal to the sagittal plane in the head.

- The pairs of canals function as a gauge of rotatory acceleration and react to the rotational movements of the head in the corresponding plane.
- The otoliths function as a gauge of gravity and linear acceleration.

1.3   Peripheral versus Central Vestibular Forms of Vertigo

The most frequent forms of peripheral vestibular vertigo are:

- Benign paroxysmal positioning vertigo (BPPV)
- Menière's disease
- Vestibular neuritis

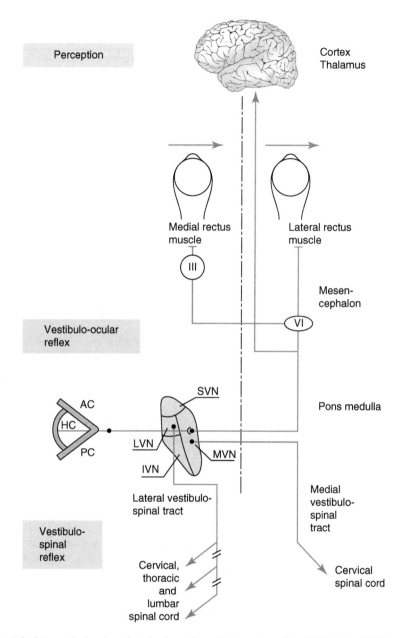

Fig. 1.2 Schematic drawing of the horizontal vestibulo-ocular reflex (VOR). The VOR is a part of a complex sensorimotor system, which makes possible perception of head position and motion (connections via the thalamus to the vestibular cortex), gaze stability (three-neuron arc to the nuclei of the ocular muscles), as well as head and postural control (vestibulo-spinal reflexes). *AC, HC, PC* anterior, horizontal, and posterior semicircular canals; *SVN, LVN, IVN, MVN* superior, lateral, inferior, and medial vestibular nuclei; and *III, VI* oculomotor and abducens nuclei

Table 1.1 Relative frequency of different vertigo syndromes diagnosed in our interdisciplinary special outpatient clinic for dizziness ($n = 14,790$ patients)

Vertigo syndromes	Frequency	
	n	%
Benign paroxysmal positioning vertigo	2,618	17.7
Somatoform phobic postural vertigo	2,157	14.6
Central vestibular vertigo	1,798	12.2
Vestibular migraine	1,662	11.2
Menière's disease	1,490	10.1
Vestibular neuritis	1,198	8.1
Bilateral vestibulopathy	1,067	7.2
Vestibular paroxysmia	569	3.9
Other psychogenic forms of vertigo	453	3.1
Perilymph fistula	83	0.6
Unclear vertigo syndromes	408	2.8
Other disorders[a]	1,287	8.8
Total number of patients	14,790	

[a]Other disorders are, for example, non-vestibular vertigo in neurodegenerative diseases or non-vestibular ocular motor disorders in myasthenia gravis or peripheral ocular motor palsies

Bilateral vestibulopathy, vestibular paroxysmia (the neurovascular compression syndrome of the eighth cranial nerve), and perilymph fistulas are more rare (Table 1.1). Acute peripheral vestibular dysfunction is—as a rule—characterized by an acute strong rotatory vertigo and peripheral vestibular spontaneous nystagmus in one direction, a tendency to fall in the other direction as well as nausea and vomiting.

Central vestibular forms of vertigo arise from lesions in the brainstem or vestibulocerebellum or of the connections between both as well as those between the vestibular nuclei and the vestibular/ocular motor structures of the brainstem, thalamus, and vestibular cortex:

- On the one hand, these are clearly defined clinical syndromes of various etiologies, for example, downbeat or upbeat nystagmus (the quick phase of nystagmus beats downward or upward). The occurrence of these typical ocular motor findings in only the cerebellar or brainstem lesions allows their definitive localization.
- On the other hand, central vestibular vertigo can also be a part of a more complex infratentorial clinical syndrome with other symptoms or supranuclear/nuclear/fascicular ocular motor disorders and/or other neurological brainstem deficits (e.g., in Wallenberg's syndrome or midbrain infarction).

Central forms of vertigo can manifest as attacks lasting for seconds or minutes (paroxysmal brainstem attacks, vestibular migraine), for hours or up to days (vestibular migraine, episodic ataxia type 2), or as a permanent syndrome (downbeat nystagmus syndrome in cases of degenerative cerebellar diseases).

1.4   The Frequency of Various Forms of Vertigo

The following relative frequencies of individual diagnoses are reported in a multiregional interdisciplinary outpatient clinic for dizziness as follows (Table 1.1). BPPV is the most frequent cause, occurring in 17.7 % of the patients. The second most frequent diagnosis is phobic postural vertigo (14.6 %) (the most frequent form of dizziness in young adults), followed by central forms of vestibular vertigo in primarily vascular and inflammatory diseases (multiple sclerosis plaques) and neurodegenerative diseases of the cerebellum or brainstem. Vestibular migraine is the most frequent cause of spontaneously recurring attacks of vertigo (11.2 %). It has one frequency peak in the second decade and another in the sixth decade; thus, it is by no means only a disease of younger women. As regards total frequency, it now takes the fourth place followed by Menière's disease and vestibular neuritis. Bilateral vestibulopathy is characterized by movement-dependent postural imbalance, is frequently not diagnosed, and occurs very often in patients of advanced age. More seldom are vestibular paroxysmia and perilymph fistula with its most frequent form superior canal dehiscence syndrome (SCDS).

It is difficult to compare the frequency data of various hospitals and medical specializations, because the definitions of the term and concept "vertigo/dizziness" differ greatly. Some are broader, others more narrow. Vertigo/dizziness is seen either as a subjective symptom or as a vestibular disorder that can be objectified. Both tendencies are dissatisfying, as the symptom of vertigo/dizziness is, on the one hand, observed in non-vestibular disturbances (e.g., orthostatic dysregulation) and, on the other, central vestibular disturbances (e.g., lateropulsion in Wallenberg's syndrome or thalamic astasia) may also occur without any subjective dizziness.

Vertigo/dizziness is also frequently seen in emergency situations. A retrospective study of more than 4,000 consecutive emergency neurological consultations in 1 year reported that headache (21 %) was the most frequent cardinal symptom, followed by motor deficit (13 %), dizziness (12 %), and epileptic attack (11 %) (Royl et al. 2010). In an emergency situation, one must first and foremost quickly differentiate between central and peripheral causes (Cnyrim et al. 2008), since this has immediate diagnostic and therapeutic consequences.

1.5   Patient History

Vertigo—in the pathological sense—is considered either an unpleasant disturbance of spatial orientation or the illusory perception of a movement of the body (spinning and wobbling) and/or of the surroundings. Care is necessary when taking the neuro-otological history of the patient (the usual pre-prepared vertigo questionnaire cannot replace it), especially because the patient's complaint of being "dizzy" is ambiguous. The important criteria for differentiating the various dizziness/vertigo syndromes, also the basis for clinical classification (Bisdorff et al. 2009), are as follows.

Table 1.2 Vertigo as light-headedness (causes given in alphabetical order)

Presyncopal light-headedness
Cardiac arrhythmia and other heart diseases
Neurocardiogenic (pre-)syncope
Orthostatic dysregulation
Vasovagal attacks
Psychiatric/psychosomatic/somatoform illnesses
Acrophobia
Agoraphobia
Hyperventilation syndrome
Panic attacks
Phobic postural vertigo
Metabolic disorders and exogenic noxious agents
Alcohol
Electrolyte disorders (hypercalcemia, hyponatremia)
Hypoglycemia
Intoxications
Medications (see Table 6.3)
Toxic substances

1.5.1   Criteria for Differentiating the Vertigo Syndromes

1.5.1.1   Type of Vertigo

To determine the type of vertigo and dizziness, it is necessary to provide the patient with comparisons. For example:

- Rotatory vertigo as when riding a merry-go-round (e.g., acute vestibular neuritis)
- Postural imbalance, as during boat trips (e.g., bilateral vestibulopathy)
- Light-headedness (e.g., phobic postural vertigo or drug intoxication) (Table 1.2)

1.5.1.2   Duration of Vertigo

If a patient has attacks of vertigo, it is important to define the minimal and maximal duration of the attacks. Examples are:

- Attacks of vertigo that last for seconds to minutes (vestibular paroxysmia)
- Attacks lasting over many minutes to hours (e.g., Menière's disease, vestibular migraine, or transient ischemic attack of the brainstem; Table 1.3)
- Persistent vertigo lasting for many days to a few weeks (e.g., acute vestibular neuritis)
- Postural imbalance lasting for years (e.g., phobic postural vertigo, bilateral vestibulopathy, or downbeat nystagmus syndrome; Table 1.4)

Table 1.3 Episodic vertigo, diseases with recurrent attacks of vertigo

Labyrinth/vestibulocochlear nerve

Benign paroxysmal positioning vertigo (only during changes of head position)

Cogan's syndrome

Menière's disease

Perilymph fistula in particular SCDS (symptoms induced by coughing, pressing, or loud sounds of a specific frequency, i.e., Tullio phenomenon)

Tumors of the cerebellopontine angle

Vestibular paroxysmia

Central vestibular system

Episodic ataxia type 2

Paroxysmal ataxia/dysarthrophonia (multiple sclerosis)

Paroxysmal ocular tilt reaction

Room-tilt illusion

Rotational vertebral artery occlusion syndrome

Transient vertebrobasilar ischemia

Vestibular epilepsy

Peripheral and/or central

Benign paroxysmal vertigo of childhood

Vertebrobasilar transient ischemia (e.g., anterior inferior cerebellar artery)

Vestibular migraine

Table 1.4 Persistent rotatory vertigo or prolonged postural vertigo

Viral infections

Herpes zoster oticus

Vestibular neuritis (herpes simplex virus type 1)

Viral neurolabyrinthitis

Bacterial infections

Meningitis

Cholesteatoma

Otitis media (direct or indirect)

Tuberculous labyrinthitis

Autoimmunological inner-ear diseases (see Table 2.4)

Tumors

Epidermoid cyst

Glomus tumor

Meningioma

Meningeosis carcinomatosa

Metastasis

Vestibular schwannoma unilateral or bilateral (as in neurofibromatosis type 2)

Vascular

Labyrinthine infarction (anterior inferior cerebellar artery or A. labyrinthi)

Pontomedullary brainstem infarction or cerebellar infarction

(continued)

Table 1.4 (continued)

Vertebrobasilar ectasia
Traumatic
Labyrinthine concussion
Petrous bone fracture (transverse > longitudinal fracture)
Brainstem concussion
Perilymph fistula
Posttraumatic otolith vertigo
Iatrogenic
Aminoglycosides (systemic or local)
Other ototoxic substances (see Table 2.4)
Temporal bone/ear surgery

Table 1.5 Causes of vertigo triggered by lateral (horizontal) head rotation in an upright position

Hypersensitive carotid sinus syndrome
Rotational vertebral artery occlusion syndrome
Compression of the eighth nerve due to cerebellopontine angle mass
Vestibular paroxysmia

1.5.1.3 Trigger/Exacerbation/Improvement of Vertigo

These features of the disorder must be explicitly asked of the patient, for example, vertigo or dizziness:

- Already at rest (e.g., acute vestibular neuritis, downbeat nystagmus syndrome, attacks of vestibular migraine, or Menière's disease)
- While walking (e.g., bilateral vestibulopathy)
- While turning the head to the side (e.g., bilateral vestibulopathy, vestibular paroxysmia, Table 1.5)
- When changing head position relative to gravity (e.g., BPPV)
- When coughing, pressing, or at loud sounds of a certain frequency—as the Tullio phenomenon (e.g., perilymph fistula, SCDS)
- Context-dependent intensity (worsening in certain social or environmental situations with improvement during sport activities or after light alcoholic drinks, e.g., phobic postural vertigo)

1.5.1.4 Accompanying Symptoms

Any further questions should aim to identify possible accompanying symptoms. Here too it is necessary to investigate each possible symptom individually:

- Accompanying symptoms can originate, on the one hand, from the inner ear, as, for example, hearing loss, tinnitus, or a feeling of pressure in one of the ears as in Menière's disease.

- On the other hand, they can originate from the brainstem or cerebellum, as, for example, double vision, perioral paresthesia, disorders of swallowing or speaking, impaired sensation of the arms or legs, or ataxia.
- Finally, migraine-typical symptoms can occur like headache and light and noise sensitivity, which suggest vestibular migraine.

The accompanying symptoms can be grouped individually by their respective causes (in alphabetical order) as follows:

Combination of Vestibular and Audiological Symptoms

- Cerebellopontine angle tumor
- Cholesteatoma
- Cogan's syndrome or other autoimmune diseases
- Ear/head trauma (labyrinthine concussion)
- Inner-ear malformation
- Labyrinthine infarct (anterior inferior cerebellar artery, labyrinthine artery)
- Menière's disease
- Neurolabyrinthitis
- Otosclerosis
- Perilymph fistula/SCDS
- Pontomedullary brainstem infarct
- Pontomedullary MS plaque
- Vestibular paroxysmia
- Zoster oticus

Illusionary Movements of the Surroundings (Oscillopsia) with Head Stationary

- Acquired fixation/pendular nystagmus
- Congenital/infantile nystagmus (depending on direction of gaze)
- Convergence–retraction nystagmus
- Downbeat nystagmus
- Myokymia of the superior oblique muscle (monocular oscillopsia)
- Ocular flutter
- Opsoclonus
- Paroxysmal ocular tilt reaction
- Peripheral vestibular spontaneous nystagmus
- Periodic alternating nystagmus
- Spasmus nutans (children)
- Upbeat nystagmus
- Vestibular paroxysmia
- Voluntary nystagmus

Only During Head Movements

- Bilateral vestibulopathy
- BPPV
- Central positional/positioning nystagmus
- Intoxication (e.g., anticonvulsants, alcohol-induced positional nystagmus)
- Perilymph fistulas/SCDS
- Peripheral or central ocular motor disorders
- Posttraumatic otolith vertigo
- Rotational vertebral artery occlusion syndrome (during head rotation)
- Vestibular paroxysmia (only in some patients)
- Vestibulocerebellar ataxia

Vertigo with Additional Brainstem/Cerebellar Symptoms

- Brainstem encephalitis
- Cerebellitis
- Craniocervical malformations (e.g., Arnold–Chiari malformation)
- Episodic ataxia type 2
- Hemorrhages (e.g., cavernoma)
- Head trauma
- Inflammation (e.g., MS plaque)
- Intoxication
- Lacunar or territorial infarcts
- Tumors of the cerebellopontine angle, brainstem, or cerebellum
- Vestibular migraine

Vertigo with Headache

- Brainstem/cerebellar ischemia
- Head trauma (especially transverse temporal bone fracture)
- Infratentorial hemorrhage
- Infratentorial tumor
- Inner-/middle-ear infections
- Vertebrobasilar dissection
- Vestibular migraine
- Zoster oticus

Vertigo with Impaired Stance and Gait

In many cases, the analysis of the control of stance, posture, and gait allows differentiation between peripheral (Table 1.6) and central vestibular (Table 1.7) disorders.

Table 1.6 Disturbances of posture and gait control in peripheral vestibular disorders

Illness	Direction of deviation	Pathomechanism
Acute vestibular neuritis	Ipsiversive	Vestibular tonus imbalance due to failure of the horizontal and anterior semicircular canal and utricle
Benign paroxysmal positioning vertigo (during changes in head position)	Forward and ipsiversive	Ampullofugal stimulation of the posterior canal due to canalolithiasis that leads to endolymph flow
Attacks of Menière's disease (Tumarkin's otolithic crisis)	Lateral, ipsiversive, or contraversive (sudden falls)	Variations of the endolymph pressure lead to an abnormal stimulation or inhibition of the otoliths and sudden vestibulospinal tonus failure
Tullio phenomenon	Backward, contraversive, diagonal	Stimulation of the otoliths by sounds of certain frequencies, e.g., in cases of perilymph fistulas
Vestibular paroxysmia	Contraversive or in different directions	Neurovascular compression of the vestibulocochlear nerve and excitation (rarely inhibition) of the vestibular nerve
Bilateral vestibulopathy	Different directions	Failure of vestibulospinal postural reflexes, exacerbated in the dark and on uneven ground

Table 1.7 Disturbance of posture and gait control in central vestibular disorders

Illness	Direction of deviation	Pathomechanism
Vestibular epilepsy (rare)	Contraversive	Focal seizures due to epileptic discharges of the vestibular cortex
Thalamic astasia (often overlooked)	Contraversive or ipsiversive	Vestibular tonus imbalance due to lesions of the posterolateral thalamus
Ocular tilt reaction (OTR)	Contraversive with mesencephalic lesions, ipsiversive with pontomedullary lesions, ipsi- or contraversive with unilateral cerebellar lesions (uvula or dentate nucleus)	Tonus imbalance of the VOR in the roll plane with lesions of the vertical canal or otolith pathways
Paroxysmal ocular tilt reaction	Ipsiversive with mesencephalic excitation, contraversive with pontomedullary excitation or excitation of the vestibular nerve	Pathological excitation of the otolith or vertical canal pathways (VOR in the roll plane)
Lateropulsion (Wallenberg's syndrome)	Ipsiversive, diagonal	Central vestibular tonus imbalance (roll and yaw planes) with tilt of subjective vertical
Downbeat nystagmus syndrome	Backward	Vestibular tonus imbalance in the pitch plane

1.6   Neuro-ophthalmological and Neuro-otological Examination

Besides the detailed patient history, which is the key to diagnosis, the systematic neuro-ophthalmological and neuro-otological examinations are especially impor- tant. In the clinical examination, the physician should at first try to differentiate between peripheral vestibular and central vestibular forms of vertigo as well as between peripheral and central ocular motor disorders. This has immediate diagnos- tic and therapeutic consequences especially in cases of acute symptoms. The fol- lowing aspects of the physical examination of patients with vertigo are obligatory:

- *Examine the eye position during straight-ahead gaze*, especially as regards verti- cal divergence (the so-called skew deviation; one eye is higher than the other) as part of the so-called ocular tilt reaction (OTR).
- *Examine the patient for nystagmus*. It is important to use Frenzel's glasses, in particular to differentiate between a peripheral vestibular spontaneous nystag- mus that can be suppressed by visual fixation and a central fixation nystagmus; the latter is typically also present during fixation or is even intensified by it.
- *Examine the different types of eye movements* (especially smooth pursuit, sac- cades, gaze-holding function) for central eye movement disorders such as sac- cadic smooth pursuit, gaze palsy, gaze-evoked nystagmus, disorder of saccades as well as impaired visual fixation suppression of the VOR. If patients with acute vertigo have central ocular motor disorders, this suggests a central origin, as, for example, an ischemia or inflammation in the area of the brainstem or cerebellum.
- *Perform the head-impulse test according to Halmagyi–Curthoys*, addressing the question of a unilateral or bilateral functional deficit of the VOR (Halmagyi and Curthoys 1988). If the patient has an acute vertigo with nystagmus but the head-impulse test does not give a pathological result, this indicates it has a central origin (Newman-Toker et al. 2008).
- *Perform positioning maneuver* to determine if there is a positioning nystagmus or positioning vertigo, also to differentiate between a BPPV and a central posi- tional or positioning nystagmus.
- *Determine the subjective visual vertical* (*SVV*) using the so-called bucket test (Zwergal et al. 2009). A deviation of the SVV occurs in more than 90 % of all acute unilateral peripheral and central vestibular disorders. It is thus a very sensi- tive sign that can be readily examined in the office using the bucket test, but it does not differentiate between a central or peripheral vestibular lesion.
- *Examine patient's hearing.*
- *Examine patient's stance and gait with the eyes open and closed.*

1.6.1   The Examination Procedure

Table 1.8 and Figs. 1.3, 1.4, 1.5, 1.6, 1.7, 1.8, 1.9, 1.10, 1.11, 1.12, 1.13, 1.14, 1.15, 1.16, 1.17, and 1.18 illustrate the individual examination procedures, the essential

Table 1.8 Examination procedures for ocular motor and vestibular systems

Type of examination	Question
Inspection	
Head/body posture	Tilt or turn of head/body
Position of eyelids	Ptosis
Eye position/motility (http://extra.springer.com)	
Position of eyes during straight-ahead gaze	Misalignment in primary position, spontaneous or fixation nystagmus
Cover/uncover test	Horizontal or vertical misalignment
Examination of eyes in eight positions (binocular and monocular)	Determination of range of motility, gaze-evoked nystagmus, end-position nystagmus
Gaze-holding function (http://extra.springer.com)	
10–40° in the horizontal or 10–20° in the vertical and back to 0°	Gaze-evoked nystagmus (http://extra.springer.com): horizontal and vertical, rebound nystagmus (http://extra.springer.com)
Slow smooth pursuit movements (http://extra.springer.com)	
Horizontal and vertical	Smooth or saccadic
Saccades (http://extra.springer.com)	
Horizontal and vertical when looking around or at targets	Latency, velocity, accuracy, conjugacy
Optokinetic nystagmus (OKN)	
Horizontal and vertical with OKN drum or tape	Inducible, direction, phase (reversal or monocularly diagonal)
Peripheral vestibular function	
Head-impulse test for clinical examination of the VOR (http://extra.springer.com) (Halmagyi–Curthoys test): rapid turning of the head and fixation of a stationary target	Unilateral or bilateral peripheral vestibular deficit
Fixation suppression of the VOR	
Turning the head and fixation of a target moving at same speed	Impairment of fixation suppression of the VOR
Examination with Frenzel's glasses	
Straight-ahead gaze, to the right, to the left, downward, and upward	Peripheral vestibular spontaneous nystagmus (http://extra.springer.com) versus central fixation nystagmus
Head-shaking test (http://extra.springer.com)	Head-shaking nystagmus
Positioning maneuver (with Frenzel's glasses) (http://extra.springer.com)	
To the right, left, head-hanging position, turning about the cephalocaudal axis	Peripheral or central positional or positioning nystagmus
Posture and balance control	
Romberg's test and simple/difficult posture and gait tests	Instability, tendency to fall
Open–closed eyes	
With/without reclining the head	
With/without distraction (writing numbers on the skin, doing maths mentally)	Psychogenic etiology

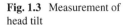

Fig. 1.3 Measurement of
head tilt

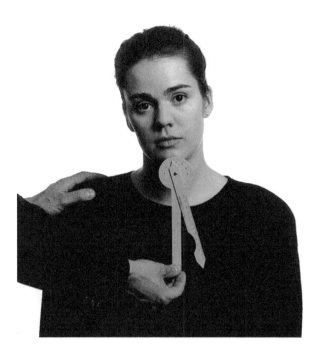

findings, and their interpretation. If the patient history and physical examination have been done carefully and systematically, additional laboratory and imaging examinations are in many cases of minor clinical significance.

1.6.1.1   Measurement of Head Tilt (Fig. 1.3)

An abnormal position of the head toward the right or left shoulder is especially observed in patients with paresis of the oblique eye muscles (e.g., palsy of the trochlear nerve or the superior oblique muscle, in which the head is turned to the non-affected side to lessen diplopia) or in those with an ocular tilt reaction (http://extra.springer.com) due to a tonus imbalance of the VOR in the roll plane. In the OTR, the head is tilted to the side of the lower eye.

A tilting of the head to the side of the lesion indicates either an acute unilateral peripheral vestibular lesion or an acute unilateral central lesion in the medulla oblongata (e.g., in Wallenberg's syndrome); a head tilt to the contralateral side occurs in pontomesencephalic lesions.

1.6.1.2   The Cover Tests (Fig. 1.4)

These tests allow diagnosis of a latent or manifest strabismus. The prerequisite for all cover tests is the presence of foveal fixation.

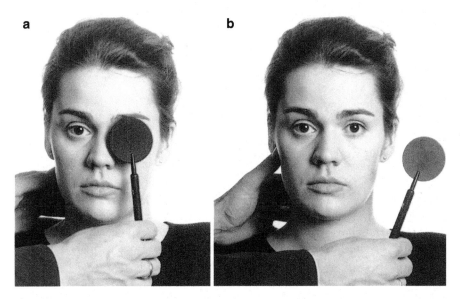

Fig. 1.4 (**a**) Cover test and (**b**) uncover test: examination for detecting misalignments of the visual axes

The One-Eye Cover Test (Fig. 1.4a)

In the one-eye cover test (http://extra.springer.com), the presence of a so-called heterotropia (i.e., manifest strabismus) can be observed in the uncovered eye; the latter moves when the other eye is covered. Heterotropia is defined as a misalignment of the visual axes, even during binocular fixation.

First, the patient is asked to fixate either a near target (at a distance of 30–40 cm) or one 5–6 m away. Then the examiner covers one eye and looks for correction movements of the now uncovered eye. If the uncovered eye moves:

- From the inside outward, esotropia is present.
- From the outside inward, exotropia.
- From above downward, hypertropia.
- From below upward, hypotropia.

  Then the other eye is examined.

The Cover/Uncover Test (Fig. 1.4b)

The one-eye cover/uncover test (http://extra.springer.com) is used to prove the presence of a heterophoria (i.e., latent strabismus). This is a misalignment of the eye axes when a target is fixated with one eye only. It is important to perform the above-mentioned cover part of the test before the cover/uncover part in order to exclude first of all a heterotropia.

First, one eye is covered for about 10 s, then uncovered; the possible corrective movements of the previously covered eye are observed. If it moves:

- Outside, esophoria is present.
- Inside, an exophoria.
- Downward, a hyperphoria.
- Upward, a hypophoria.

The Alternating Cover Test

This test (http://extra.springer.com) is also useful for determining the maximal misalignment of the eye axes in both a tropia and a phoria. The alternating cover test is also helpful when establishing a vertical divergence/skew deviation (in the context of an OTR) (http://extra.springer.com), i.e., a vertical misalignment of the eyes that cannot be explained by an ocular muscle palsy or damage of a peripheral nerve. It is necessary to look for vertical corrective movements, when the cover is switched from one eye to the other. In contrast to trochlear nerve palsy or superior oblique muscle palsy, in skew deviation as a component of the OTR, the vertical misalignment changes little or not at all during different directions of gaze.

1.6.1.3 Examination of the Eyes: Gaze Positions (Fig. 1.5)

In the clinical examination of the eyes in nine different positions (http://extra. springer.com), it is necessary to look for:

- Misalignment of the axes of the eyes (see above)
- Fixation disorders
- Peripheral vestibular spontaneous nystagmus and central fixation nystagmus
- The range of eye movements
- Gaze-evoked nystagmus, i.e., disorders of the gaze-holding function

The examination can be performed with an object for fixation or a small rod-shaped flashlight. In the primary position, one should first look for misalignment of the axes of the eyes and periodic eye movements, especially spontaneous nystagmus or so-called saccadic oscillations/intrusions:

- Horizontal rotatory (typical for an acute vestibular neuritis).
- Beating vertically upward or downward (downbeat, upbeat nystagmus syndrome) (http://extra.springer.com).
- Suppression of the nytagmus by visual fixation (typical for peripheral vestibular spontaneous nystagmus (see below)).
- During fixation only slight suppression (or even increase) of intensity of the nystagmus (typical for central fixation nystagmus). A congenital nystagmus (http://extra.springer.com) beats horizontally as a rule at various frequencies and amplitudes and increases during fixation.

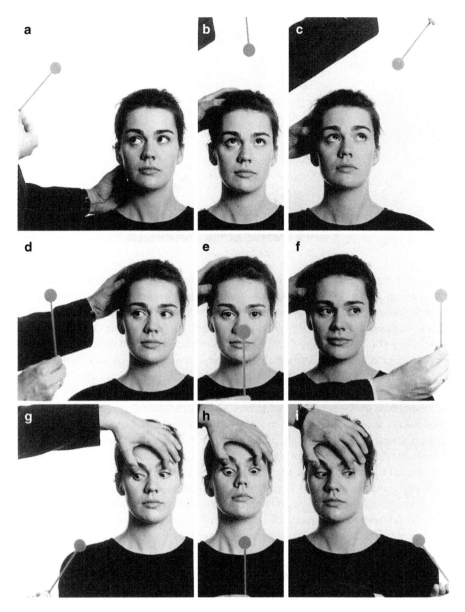

Fig. 1.5 (a–i) Examination of the eyes in nine different positions

So-called square-wave jerks (http://extra.springer.com) (small saccades of 0.5–5° with an intersaccadic interval) cause the eyes to oscillate around the primary position and are observed in progressive supranuclear palsy or certain cerebellar syndromes.

Fig. 1.6 Clinical examination of eye positions and eye movements with an examination flashlight

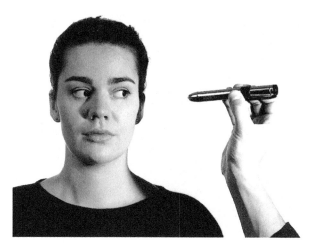

Ocular flutter (intermittent rapid bursts of horizontal oscillations without an intersaccadic interval) or opsoclonus (http://extra.springer.com) (combined horizontal, vertical, and torsional oscillations also without an intersaccadic interval) is in a strict sense not a form of nystagmus but the so-called saccadic oscillation/intrusion. They occur in various disorders, for example, in encephalitis, tumors of the brainstem or cerebellum, intoxication, or most often in paraneoplastic syndromes.

After checking for a possible misalignment of the axes of the eyes (see cover test) (http://extra.springer.com) and possible eye movements in primary position (spontaneous nystagmus), the examiner should then establish the range of eye movements monocularly and binocularly in the eight end positions (Fig. 1.5); deficits found here can as a rule indicate ocular muscle or nerve palsy. Moreover, a gaze-evoked nystagmus (gaze-holding deficit) (http://extra.springer.com) can be determined by examining the eccentric gaze positions.

Using a small rod-shaped flashlight (Fig. 1.6) has the advantage that the corneal reflex images can be observed and thus ocular misalignments can be easily detected. Note: It is important to observe the corneal reflex images from the direction of the illumination and to ensure that the patient attentively fixates the object.

Examination for a Gaze-Holding Deficit

Gaze-evoked nystagmus often allows a topographical-anatomical diagnosis:

- A gaze-evoked nystagmus in all directions occurs in cerebellar disorders (especially impaired function of the flocculus/paraflocculus), above all in neurodegenerative diseases, but can also be caused by drugs (e.g., anticonvulsants, benzodiazepines) or alcohol.
- A purely horizontal gaze-evoked nystagmus can indicate a structural lesion in the area of the brainstem (nucleus prepositus hypoglossi, vestibular nuclei) and cerebellum (flocculus/paraflocculus), i.e., the neural integrator for horizontal gaze-holding function.

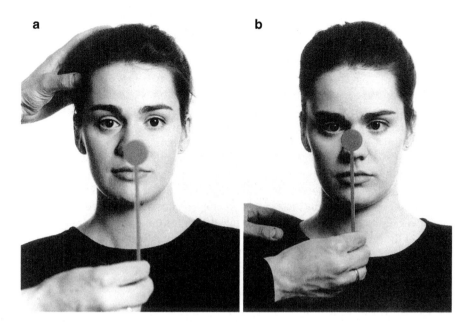

Fig. 1.7 (**a**) Vergence test and (**b**) convergence reaction

- A purely vertical gaze-evoked nystagmus is observed in midbrain lesions involving the interstitial nucleus of Cajal (INC), i.e., the neural integrator for vertical gaze-holding function.
- A dissociated horizontal gaze-evoked nystagmus (greater in the abducting than the adducting eye) in combination with an adduction deficit are the signs of internuclear ophthalmoplegia (INO) due to a defect of the medial longitudinal fascicle (MLF), ipsilateral to the adduction deficit.
- Downbeat nystagmus (http://extra.springer.com) usually increases when looking down and especially to the side. A nystagmus beating diagonally and downward is found in the sideward gaze. The cause of downbeat nystagmus is generally a bilaterally impaired function of the flocculus/paraflocculus.
- To examine for a so-called rebound nystagmus (http://extra.springer.com), the patient should gaze for at least 60s to one side and then return the eyes to the primary position; this can cause a transient nystagmus to appear with slow phases in the direction of the previous eye position. Rebound nystagmus generally indicates damage of the flocculus/paraflocculus or cerebellar pathways.

1.6.1.4   Vergence Test and Convergence Reaction (Fig. 1.7)

A target is moved from a distance of about 50 cm toward the patient's eyes, or the patient looks back and forth between a distant and a near target. Looking nearby causes vergence, accommodation, and miosis, i.e., the convergence reaction. Neurons important for the convergence reaction are in the area of the mesencephalic reticular formation and the oculomotor nucleus. This explains why the convergence reaction is disturbed in rostral midbrain lesions and tumors of the pineal region and thalamus and why abnormalities of vertical gaze are often associated with these defects. In certain neurodegenerative disorders such as progressive supranuclear palsy (http://extra. springer.com), convergence is also often impaired. Inborn defects of the convergence reaction (http://extra.springer.com) also occur in some forms of strabismus.

Convergence–retraction nystagmus can be induced by having the patient look upward and having him make saccades vertically upward or look at a moving optokinetic drum with its stripes going downward. Instead of vertical saccades, rapid, convergent eye movements result that are associated with retractions of the eyeball. The site of damage is the posterior commissure or in rare cases a bilateral disorder of the rostral interstitial nucleus of medial longitudinal fasciculus (riMLF).

A spasm of the near reflex is a voluntary convergence accompanied by pupillary constriction; the latter is an important clinical sign for the diagnosis. Occasionally spasm of the near reflex is psychogenic. It can mimic bilateral abducens palsy.

1.6.1.5 Clinical Examination of Saccades (Fig. 1.8)

First, it is necessary to observe spontaneous saccades triggered by visual or auditory stimuli. Then the patient is asked to glance back and forth between two horizontal or two vertical targets. The velocity, accuracy, and the conjugacy of the saccades should be noted:

- Normal individuals can immediately reach the target with a single fast movement or one small corrective saccade.
- Slowing of saccades in all directions (http://extra.springer.com)—often accompanied by hypometric saccades (http://extra.springer.com)—occurs, for example, in neurodegenerative disorders or with intoxication (medication, especially anticonvulsants or benzodiazepines).
- Isolated slowing of horizontal saccades (http://extra.springer.com) is observed in pontine brainstem lesions due to a dysfunction of the ipsilateral paramedian pontine reticular formation (PPRF).
- Isolated slowing of vertical saccades (http://extra.springer.com) indicates a midbrain lesion in which the rostral interstitial medial longitudinal fascicle (riMLF) is involved, in fact in ischemic or neurodegenerative diseases, especially progressive supranuclear palsy.
- Hypermetric saccades (http://extra.springer.com), which can be identified by a corrective saccade back to the object, indicate lesions of the cerebellum (especially the vermis) or the cerebellar pathways.
- Patients with Wallenberg's syndrome (http://extra.springer.com) make hypermetric saccades toward the side of the lesion and hypometric saccades toward the opposite side due to a dysfunction of the inferior cerebellar peduncle; defects of the superior cerebellar peduncle, conversely, lead to contralateral hypermetric saccades.

Fig. 1.8 (**a, b**) Clinical
examination of saccades

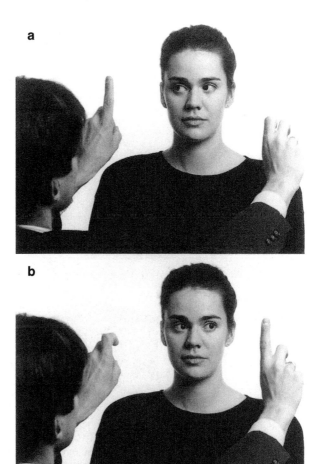

- A slowing of the adducting saccade ipsilateral to a lesion of the MLF (http://
  extra.springer.com) is pathognomonic for internuclear ophthalmoplegia (INO).
- Delayed initiation of saccades is most often due to supratentorial cortical dysfunction, affecting the frontal or parietal eye field (e.g., Balint's syndrome).

1.6.1.6   Clinical Examination of Smooth Pursuit Eye Movements (Fig. 1.9)

The generation of smooth pursuit eye movements (http://extra.springer.com),
which keep the image of an object stable on the fovea, involves diverse anatomical
structures: the visual cortex, medial temporal area, medial superior temporal area
(MST), frontal eyefields, dorsolateral pontine nuclei, cerebellum (flocculus), and

Fig. 1.9 Clinical examination of smooth pursuit eye movements

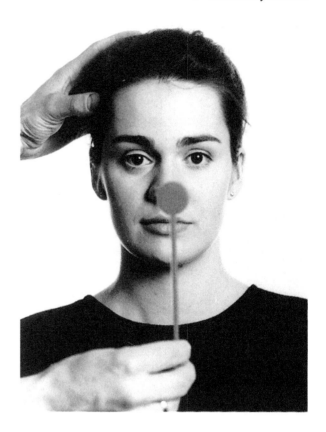

vestibular and ocular motor nuclei. These eye movements are influenced by alertness, a number of drugs, and also age. Even healthy people exhibit a slightly saccadic smooth pursuit (http://extra.springer.com) during vertical downward eye movements.

The patient is asked to track visually an object moving slowly in horizontal and vertical directions (10–20°/s) while keeping the head stationary. Corrective (catch-up or backup) saccades are looked for; they indicate a smooth pursuit gain (ratio of eye movement velocity and gaze target velocity) that is too low or too high:

- A saccadic smooth pursuit in all directions indicates an impaired function of the flocculus/paraflocculus, e.g., in spinocerebellar ataxias, drug poisoning (anticonvulsants, benzodiazepines) or alcohol.
- Marked asymmetries of smooth pursuit, however, indicate a structural lesion; if the smooth pursuit is saccaded to the left, this indicates a left-sided lesion of the flocculus/paraflocculus.
- A reversal of smooth pursuit eye movements is typical for congenital nystagmus.

Fig. 1.10 Clinical examination with Frenzel's glasses

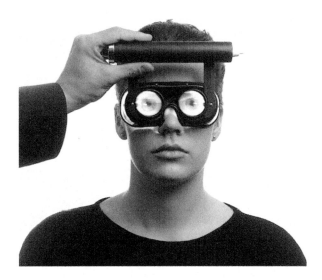

1.6.1.7 Clinical Examination with Frenzel's Glasses (Fig. 1.10)

The magnifying lenses (+16 diopters) with light inside, on the one hand, prevent visual fixation, which typically suppresses a peripheral vestibular spontaneous nystagmus and, on the other, facilitates the observation of the patient's eye movements. Examination should include:

- Peripheral vestibular spontaneous nystagmus (http://extra.springer.com).
- Head-shaking nystagmus (http://extra.springer.com) (the patient is instructed to turn his head quickly to the right and to the left about 20 times; then the eye movements are observed).
- Positioning and positional nystagmus (http://extra.springer.com).
- Hyperventilation-induced nystagmus.
- Spontaneous nystagmus indicates a tonus imbalance of the VOR; if it is caused by a peripheral vestibular lesion—as in vestibular neuritis—the nystagmus is typically dampened by visual fixation, whereas a central fixation nystagmus is not suppressed by fixation or may become even worse.
- Head-shaking nystagmus (http://extra.springer.com) is due to a latent asymmetry of the so-called velocity storage, which can be due to peripheral and central vestibular disorders. In a peripheral vestibular deficit, the head-shaking nystagmus beats toward the ear with an intact labyrinthine function. The so-called cross-coupling can occur in central cerebellar disorders: the horizontal head-shaking maneuver induces a vertical nystagmus.

1.6.1.8 Clinical Examination with Frenzel's Glasses and a Politzer Balloon (Fig. 1.11)

Changes in middle-ear pressure caused by applying pressure (either positive or negative) to the tympanic membrane with a Politzer balloon, by tragal compression,

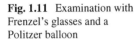

Fig. 1.11 Examination with Frenzel's glasses and a Politzer balloon

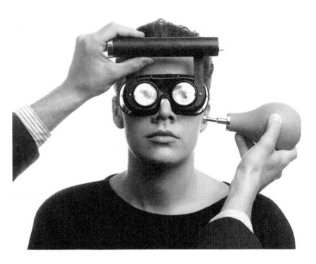

or by tones of a certain frequency or loudness (the so-called Tullio phenomenon) can induce nystagmus in patients with perilymph fistula/SCDS (http://extra. springer.com). This nystagmus—often associated with spells of vertigo and oscillopsia—can also be induced by the Valsalva maneuver, coughing, pressing, sneezing, or swallowing.

1.6.1.9 Examination with an Ophthalmoscope (Fig. 1.12)

The examination of one eye with an ophthalmoscope (DVD) while the other eye is covered is a very sensitive method for detecting nystagmus, even of minimal veloc- ity or low frequency as well as so-called square-wave jerks (http://extra.springer. com) (small saccades with an amplitude of 0.5–5° with an intersaccadic interval, that are often observed in progressive supranuclear palsy (http://extra.springer.com) or certain cerebellar syndromes). It is important to pay attention to the movements of the papilla or of the retinal blood vessels. Since the retina is behind the axis of rotation of the eyeball, the direction of any observed vertical or horizontal move- ment is opposite to that of the nystagmus, i.e., a downbeat nystagmus (http://extra. springer.com) causes a rapid upward movement of the optic papilla and retinal vessels.

1.6.1.10 Examination with the Optokinetic Drum (Fig. 1.13)

The examination of eye movements with the optokinetic drum (http://extra. springer.com) allows combined testing of smooth pursuit movements and saccades in horizontal and vertical directions. It is especially helpful with uncooperative or

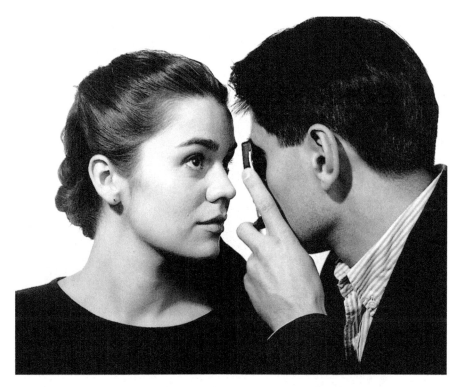

Fig. 1.12 The examination of one eye with an ophthalmoscope, a very sensitive method for detecting nystagmus. The non-examined eye should be closed to avoid visual fixation

drowsy patients as well as children. An intact horizontal and vertical optokinetic nystagmus speaks probably for intact function of the midbrain and the pons. Look for:

- Asymmetries, e.g., between right and left (indicates a unilateral cortical or pontine lesion), vertical worse than horizontal (indicative of a supranuclear gaze palsy due to a mesencephalic lesion)
- Dissociations (http://extra.springer.com) of the two eyes (a sign of diminished adduction in internuclear ophthalmoplegia)
- Reversal of pursuit (indicates congenital nystagmus) (http://extra.springer.com)

1.6.1.11 The Head-Impulse Test: Examination of the Horizontal VOR (Fig. 1.14)

To test the horizontal VOR (http://extra.springer.com), the examiner holds the patient's head between both hands, asks him to fixate a target in front of his eyes,

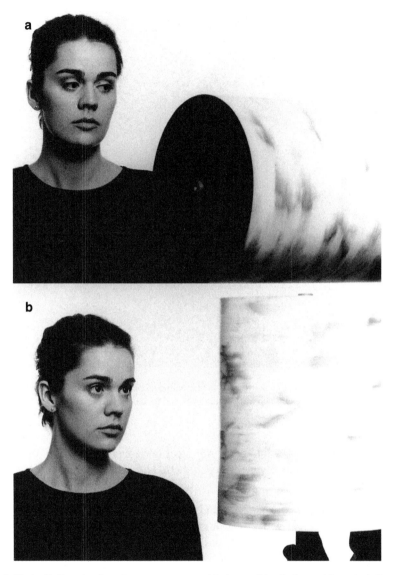

Fig. 1.13 (**a**, **b**) Examination of eye movements with the optokinetic drum: (**a**) vertical direction and (**b**) horizontal direction

and very rapidly turns the patient's head horizontally by ca. 20–30° to the right and then to the left. This is the most important bedside test for the VOR function.

• In a healthy subject, this rotation of the head causes rapid, compensatory eye movements in the opposite direction with the same angular velocity as the head movements. In this way, the target remains stable on the retina.

- In unilateral labyrinthine failure (http://extra.springer.com) (exemplified in Fig. 1.14b by failure of the right horizontal canal), the eyes move during head rotations with the head to the right, and the patient has to perform a so-called refixation saccade to the left in order to fixate the target again (Fig. 1.14b). This is the clinical sign of a deficit of the VOR (in the high-frequency range) to the right. The examination situation is shown in Fig. 1.14c.

In most cases, this test allows a clinically rapid and accurate diagnosis of a unilateral or bilateral functional disorder of the VOR. If the results are not distinct, the head-impulse test should be performed with video-oculography (Fig. 1.21). The test can also be performed in the planes of the posterior and anterior canals (with a diagonal head movement).

1.6.1.12 Testing the Visual Fixation Suppression of the VOR (Fig. 1.15)

Before performing this test, the examiner must be sure that the VOR is intact (see above). The patient is then asked to fixate a target in front of his eyes while moving his head as uniformly as possible with the same angular velocity as the target in front of the eyes, first horizontally and then vertically, back and forth at

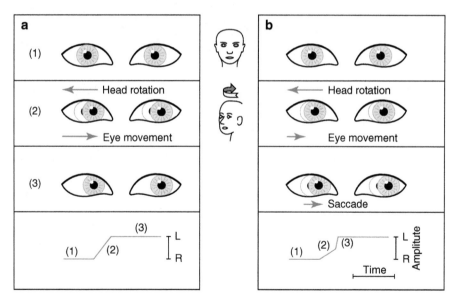

Fig. 1.14 (**a–c**) The head-impulse test: clinical examination of the horizontal vestibulo-ocular reflex (VOR) (Halmagyi and Curthoys 1988). (**a**) Normal result: The eyes move during rapid rotation of the head with the same angular velocity but in the opposite direction; thus, the eyes remain on the target. (**b**) Example: Deficit of the right horizontal semicircular canal. In cases of unilateral labyrinthine loss on the right side, the eyes move during head rotations to the right with the head, and the patient has to perform a so-called refixation saccade to the left in order to again fixate the target. This is the clinical sign of a deficit of the VOR in the high-frequency range. (**c**) The examination situation

Fig. 1.14 (continued)   c

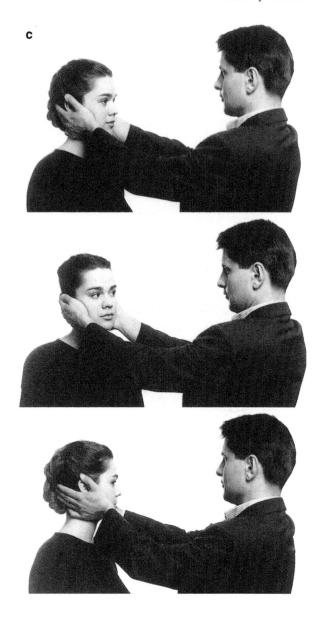

moderate speed. The examiner should watch for corrective saccades, which indicate a disorder of the visual fixation suppression of the VOR. Subsequently, the test is performed for the vertical VOR. Impaired visual fixation suppression of the VOR (http://extra.springer.com) (which as a rule occurs with smooth pursuit abnormalities, as these two functions use the same neural pathways) typically indicates lesions of the cerebellum (flocculus or paraflocculus) or of cerebellar pathways. Drugs, especially anticonvulsants and sedatives, and alcohol can also

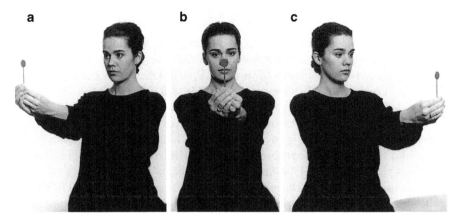

Fig. 1.15 (**a–c**) Clinical testing of visual fixation suppression of the VOR. Healthy persons can suppress the VOR by fixation. The eyes remain on the target. A minimal shift of the image on the retina (the so-called retinal slip) is the signal to suppress the VOR; this same signal is important for the smooth pursuit. The observance of saccades during this examination indicates an impairment of the smooth pursuit system, typically found in cerebellar disorders involving the flocculus or paraflocculus

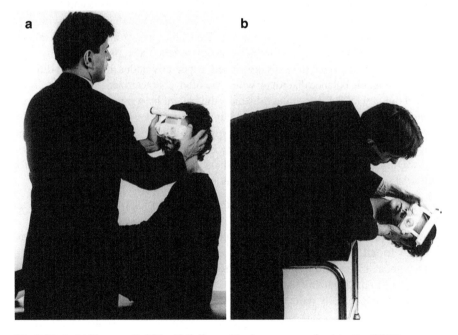

Fig. 1.16 (**a, b**) The so-called Dix–Hallpike positioning maneuver for detecting BPPV

impair visual fixation suppression of the VOR, because of their effects on the cerebellum.

1.6.1.13   The Dix–Hallpike Maneuver (Fig. 1.16)

The so-called Dix–Hallpike maneuver is performed to determine the presence of BPPV (http://extra.springer.com), generally starting from the posterior canal. While the patient is sitting, his head is first turned by 45° to one side, so that the posterior canal is parallel to the positioning plane. Then the patient is rapidly put in the supine position to the opposite side with the head hanging over the end of the examination couch.

If a BPPV of the left posterior semicircular canal, for example, is present, this maneuver will induce, with a latency of a few seconds, a crescendo–decrescendo-like nystagmus (http://extra.springer.com), which from the examiner's viewpoint rotates and beats clockwise toward the forehead. When the patient is returned to a sitting position, the nystagmus can change reverse direction. For horizontal canal BPPV, the patient's head is turned to the right and left while lying supine.

1.6.1.14   Examination of Stance (Fig. 1.17) and Gait

There are different variations and degrees of difficulty of the Romberg test: standing with feet next to each other, one foot in front of the other (tandem Romberg), or on one foot. Each variation is performed with eyes first open and then closed; with eyes closed, the visual control of the swaying during standing is examined. A peripheral vestibular functional disorder and other sensory deficits like a polyneuropathy typically cause swaying once the eyes are closed, especially under difficult conditions.

In psychogenic balance disorders, which are often characterized by a bizarre swaying without any falls, the examiner distracts the patient by writing letters or numbers on his arm or back. This reduces the swaying and indicates that the stance disorder has a psychogenic origin. Another variant of the Romberg test is standing under the above-described conditions but with head reclined backward. This generally increases the swaying. During the examination of balance under static conditions, look for increased swaying forward/backward, right/left, as well as diagonally:

- In sensory deficits (vestibular or somatosensory), closing of the eyes leads to an obvious increase in the swaying.
- A unilateral peripheral vestibular functional disorder typically leads to a tendency to fall ipsilaterally.
- Downbeat and upbeat nystagmus syndromes are associated with increased body swaying to the front and backward if eyes are closed.
- Distraction generally reduces the swaying in cases of psychogenic disorders.

When examining the patient's gait, the patient has first to go straight ahead with the eyes open then eyes closed. Subsequently, the patient has to walk on an imagined line heel to toe again with the eyes open and then closed. One has to look for step length, gait variability, and whether the gait is broad or narrow based or whether there is a deviation to the right or left. In bilateral vestibulopathy, gait is broad based and becomes worse with the eyes closed. In a unilateral peripheral vestibular loss, this also is true with a gait deviation toward the side of the vestibular lesion. With increasing speed, gait improves. In cerebellar disorders, gait is broad based with a great gait variability.

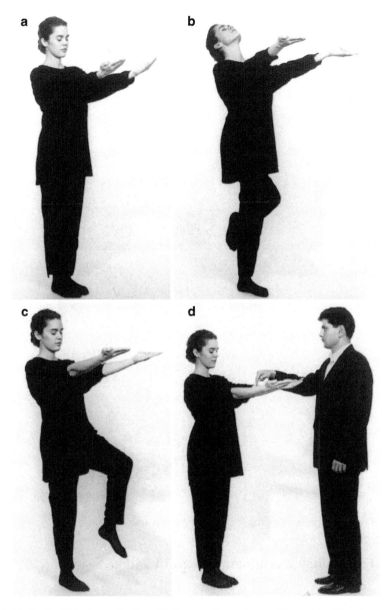

Fig. 1.17 (**a**–**d**) Clinical examination of balance under static conditions: (**a**) with eyes open and subsequently closed, (**b**) standing on one leg with head extended backward or (**c**) stepping in place, and (**d**) distracted state by writing on arm or back or by counting

1.6.1.15   Finger-Pointing Test (Fig. 1.18)

The patient is instructed to follow as precisely as possible the examiner's finger as it rapidly moves horizontally. Cerebellar ataxia is often indicated by hypermetric movements with an intention tremor. This test is more sensitive than the finger-to-nose test.

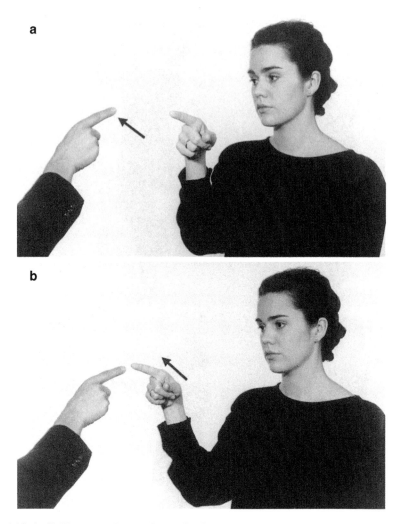

Fig. 1.18 (**a**, **b**) Finger-pointing test for ataxia of the extremities

1.7 Laboratory Examinations and Imaging

If the patient's history is taken accurately and the clinical examination is precise, laboratory examinations complement the physical examination, especially in order to quantify deficits or to document the course of the functional disorders. Table 1.9 and Figs. 1.19, 1.20, 1.21, 1.22, 1.23, 1.24, 1.25, 1.26, and 1.27 summarize the essential neuro-ophthalmological and neuro-otological procedures of examination, give typical findings, and indicate how to interpret them.

Table 1.9 Neuro-ophthalmological examination and laboratory tests for vertigo/dizziness and eye movement disorders

Technique	Features	Advantages	Disadvantages
Neuro-ophthalmological examination	Total range of eye movements, horizontal, vertical (torsional)	No technical requirements, simple, resolution <1°	No recording, eye movement velocity cannot be measured
Orthoptic examination	Fundus photography and scanning laser ophthalmoscope (SLO) (http://extra.springer.com), determination of eye misalignment and psychophysical determination of, e.g., the subjective visual vertical (http://extra.springer.com)	Precise measurement with documentation, noninvasive, well tolerated; Very sensitive for an acute unilateral vestibular lesion; cheap and easy to measure with the so-called bucket test	Expensive apparatus (e.g., scanning laser ophthalmoscope); Not specific to differentiate between a central and a peripheral lesion
Video-oculography	Measurement range ±40°, resolution of 0.1–1°	Noninvasive, well tolerated, combined with caloric testing and the head-impulse test for determining the function of the VOR; nowadays widely used	Only possible with open eyes, 3-D analysis torsion in roll plane more complicated and expensive
Electronystagmography (ENG)	Measurement range ±40°, resolution of 1°	Noninvasive, well tolerated, caloric stimulation possible	No measurement of torsional and poor measurement of vertical movements, eyelid artifacts, baseline drift
Magnetic-coil technique	Measurement range ±40°, vertical resolution of 0.02°	Best resolution of horizontal, vertical, and torsional movements (research)	Semi-invasive, unpleasant, expensive, only with cooperative patients, maximum of 30 min, local anesthesia necessary
Cervical vestibular-evoked myogenic potentials (cVEMP)	Examination of saccular function	Noninvasive, well tolerated, simple to perform	Findings in part still contradictory, in part also include the function of the vertical canals
Ocular vestibular-evoked potentials (oVEMP)	Examination of utricular function	Noninvasive, well tolerated, simple to perform	

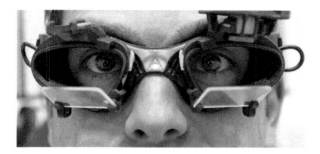

Fig. 1.19 Video-oculography (VOG) performed with a mask attached to the head in which a camera is integrated. An infrared headlight built into the mask also allows measurement of eye movements in complete darkness. The eye movements are shown online by means of a video-oculography program that continuously calculates the eye movements. Three-dimensional recordings can also be made by analyzing the movements of the picture of the iris

The four most important laboratory examinations are:

- Video-oculography (VOG) (http://extra.springer.com), including caloric testing and the head-impulse test for quantitative measurement of the VOR
- Electronystagmography (ENG) (http://extra.springer.com), which is increasingly being replaced by VOG
- Vestibular-evoked myogenic potentials (VEMP), i.e., cervical VEMP (cVEMP) for examining the saccular function and ocular VEMP (oVEMP) for examining the utricular function
- Posturography

To record eye movements for research purposes, the three-dimensional VOG or the magnetic scleral-coil technique (http://extra.springer.com) is used.

1.7.1 Video-Oculography (VOG)

Video-oculography (http://extra.springer.com) is a noninvasive method that has been so far developed over the last years that it is now used worldwide as a valid and reliable method to record eye movements. The eyes are filmed by one or two video cameras (i.e., monocular or binocular recording) integrated in a mask attached to the head (Fig. 1.19). The image of the pupils and/or light reflexes are analyzed by a computer to measure eye movements in two dimensions. This method allows rapid and reliable recording of horizontal and vertical eye movements (without muscle artifacts or unstable baseline). Recording is, however, only possible when the eyes are wide open. There is a largely linear resolution in the range of ±30°. Video-oculography is combined with caloric (Fig. 1.20) and head-impulse testing (Fig. 1.21). The 3-D representation of eye movements

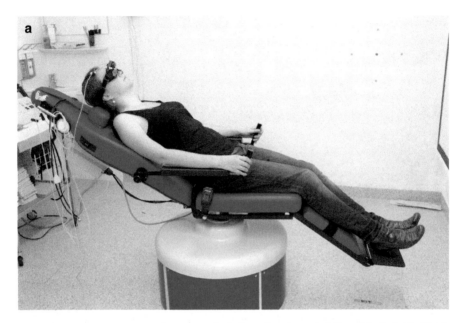

Fig. 1.20 (a, b) Caloric testing. By means of caloric testing, the excitability of the individual horizontal canals can be determined and thus whether or not they are functioning. (**a**) After excluding the possibility of a lesion of the eardrum, the head of the patient is tilted 30° upward, so that the horizontal semicircular canals approach the vertical plane. This allows optimal caloric stimulation. (**b**) The external auditory canals on each side are separately irrigated under standard conditions with 30°C cool and 44°C warm water. At the same time, the horizontal and vertical eye movements are recorded by means of video-oculography (or electronystagmography). The irrigation with 44°C warm water causes—via a combined convective and non-convective mechanism—excitation of the hair cells of the horizontal canal along with slow contraversive eye movements; 30°C cool water leads to an inhibition with slow ipsiversive eye movements. The clinically relevant parameter is the maximal velocity of the irrigation-induced eye movements (peak slow-phase velocity, PSPV); PSPV values less than 5°/s are considered pathological. Since there is considerable inter-individual variation of caloric excitability, the so-called "vestibular paresis formula" of Jongkees is used:

$$(((R30°C + R44°C) - (L30°C + L44°C)) / (R30°C + R44°C + L30°C + L44°C)) \times 100,$$

where, for instance, R30°C is the PSPV during caloric irrigation of the right ear with 30°C cool water. Values of >25 % asymmetry between the affected and non-affected ear are considered pathological and indicate, for example, a unilateral peripheral vestibular disorder

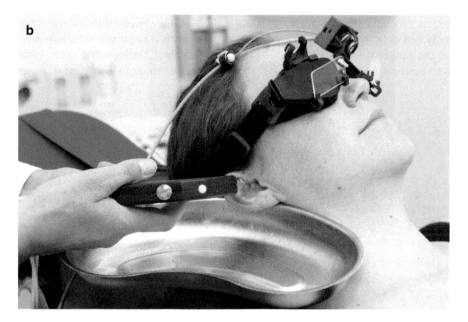

Fig. 1.20 (continued)

(i.e., additional measurement of torsion) requires an extensive analysis of the image of the iritic structures or of two additional marker dots applied to the sclera.

The VOG and simultaneous measurement of the head acceleration during the head-impulse test (Bartl et al. 2009) can be used to quantify the function of the VOR (Fig. 1.21), in particular if the results of the bedside head-impulse test are uncertain.

1.7.2   Electronystagmography (ENG)

To record eye movements quantitatively in ENG (http://extra.springer.com), two electrodes are placed horizontally and vertically on each eye so that the changes in the dipole between the retina and cornea, which occur with eye movements, can be recorded (Fig. 1.22). ENG also allows documentation of the findings (important for monitoring the course of the patient) and, for example, relatively exact measurements of saccade velocity and saccade accuracy. A rotatory chair and rotatory drum (Fig. 1.23) allow eye movements to be recorded under dynamic conditions. Irrigation of the external auditory canal with 30 °C cool and 44 °C warm water (caloric testing) can be used to identify any disturbance of peripheral vestibular function (horizontal canal).

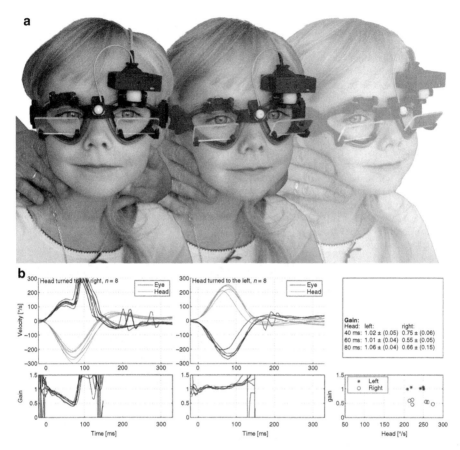

Fig. 1.21 (**a, b**) Head-impulse test with video-oculography (VOG) to quantify the function of the VOR. (**a**) The eye and head movements are simultaneously recorded. The so-called gain of the VOR can be determined from the quotients of the eye and head angular velocity. (**b**) During head impulses to the left (*right part* of Fig. b), compensatory eye movements with a similar angular velocity can be observed leading to a calculated VOR gain of about 1, indicating a normal function of the left semicircular canal. In contrast, the VOR gain during head movements to the right are reduced (*left part* of Fig. b); this indicates a right-sided peripheral vestibular deficit. Already after about 70 ms after head movement begins to the right, one can recognize correction saccades (so-called refixation saccades). In this case, these saccades would not become apparent during a clinically performed head-impulse test and are therefore called "covert saccades." They are only apparent with VOG. This means if VOG is not performed, the test results can be falsely negative

1.7.3   Neuro-orthoptic and Psychophysical Procedures

Neuro-orthoptic and psychophysical examination procedures have increasingly gained in importance in topographic diagnostics, particularly when differentiating between peripheral and central vestibular or ocular motor dysfunctions as well as

Fig. 1.22 Electronystagmography (ENG). Placement of the electrodes for monocular recording of horizontal and vertical eye movements. The electrophysiological basis of the ENG is the corneo-retinal dipole (a potential difference of about 1 μV). The dipole is parallel to the longitudinal axis of the eye, with the retina having a negative potential. Changes in this dipole between the horizontal or vertical electrodes are DC amplified. The ENG allows noninvasive horizontal recordings of ±40° with an accuracy of ca. 1° and vertical recordings of ±20°. Major disadvantages are susceptibility to eyeblink artifacts, electromyographic activity, and unstable baseline; torsional eye movements cannot be recorded with the two-dimensional ENG

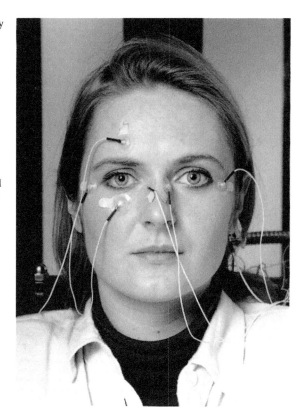

in disorders affecting areas in the brainstem and cerebellum. The following procedures are used:

- The cover and the cover/uncover test for detecting manifest and latent strabismus, in particular vertical divergence (skew deviation) (see above)
- Measurement of the range of eye movements
- Examination for central ocular motor or vestibular dysfunction
- Psychophysical determination of the subjective visual vertical (SVV) (http://extra.springer.com) (Fig. 1.24), especially with the so-called bucket test (Fig. 1.24b)
- Fundus photography or preferably the scanning laser ophthalmoscope (SLO) for measuring ocular torsion in the roll plane (see Fig. 1.25)

1.7.4   Vestibular-Evoked Myogenic Potentials (VEMP)

The function of the otolith organs can nowadays be measured with the vestibular-evoked myogenic potentials (VEMP) (Fig. 1.26): the cervical VEMP (cVEMP) are

Fig. 1.23 Electronystagmography with rotatory chair and rotatory drum (with vertical stripes) with an apparatus that projects a laser spot (above the patient). This setup allows recordings of eye movements under static conditions (e.g., test for spontaneous or gaze-evoked nystagmus, saccades, pursuit and optokinetic nystagmus) and under dynamic conditions (pre- and postrotatory nystagmus and visual fixation suppression of the VOR), as well as positional and positioning testing and caloric irrigation

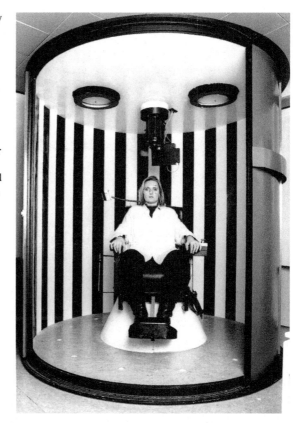

used to evaluate the function of the saccule and the ocular VEMP (oVEMP), that of the utricle (overview in Rosengren et al. 2010). It has not been conclusively clarified if these tests stimulate only the otoliths or also additionally the vertical canals. Nevertheless, the VEMP have become an important examination procedure, for until recently the function of the otolith organs could only be tested with considerable expense.

1.7.4.1   Cervical Vestibular-Evoked Myogenic Potentials (cVEMP)

The vestibulo-collic reflex is used to test the reflex arc of the saccule, which extends over the vestibular nerves, vestibular nuclei, interneurons, and motor neurons to the neck musculature (sternocleidomastoid muscles) (Fig. 1.26) (Rosengren et al. 2010). It is not necessary that hearing be preserved, since the "sensitivity to sound" or to sound waves of the saccule can be used. The prerequisite for cVEMP testing is, however, an intact middle-ear function. The reflex is triggered by a loud click or a burst. Surface EMG is used to record from both sternocleidomastoid muscles (Fig. 1.26). Healthy subjects first show on the ipsilateral side a positive wave about

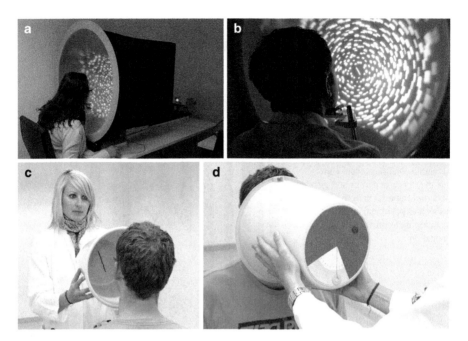

Fig. 1.24 (**a–d**) The subjective visual vertical (SVV). (**a**) For determination of the SVV, the patient sits upright in front of a hemispheric dome (60 cm in diameter) and looks into it. The dome extends beyond the limits of the patient's visual field with the result that the patient cannot orient himself spatially by fixed external structures. The hemispheric dome is illuminated with spots of light that can rotate. A short bar (14° of the visual field) is projected at the eye level of the subject. The patient should turn it by means of a potentiometer from a random initial position until he has the subjective impression that the bar is "vertical." The deviation of the bar from the objective vertical axis is measured in degrees and recorded on a PC. The mean of ten measurements equals the SVV. Under these conditions, the normal range (mean ±2 SDs) of the SVV is $0° ± 2.5°$. (**b**) Measurements can be made under static and dynamic conditions. Under dynamic conditions, the spots either rotate to the right or to the left. In addition, the measurement can be made with both eyes or each single eye. This is helpful when differentiating between central and peripheral oculomotor disorders. (**c**) A simple clinical test to determine the SVV is the so-called bucket test (modified from Zwergal et al. (2009)). The patient looks into a bucket at a line that has been drawn on the bottom and which he/she must get into a vertical position. (**d**) The examiner then reads the deviation from the actual vertical (perpendicular). This method is just as sensitive and reliable as that shown in (a)

14 s (P14) after the stimulus as well as a negative wave about 21 ms (N21) afterward (Fig. 1.26). Evaluation criteria are the presence of the waves P14 and N21 with amplitude and probably latency. Their absence as well as a clear reduction in their amplitude is considered pathological; changes in latency are apparently of inferior importance.

Pathological findings of the cVEMP were reported for the following primarily peripheral vestibular diseases:

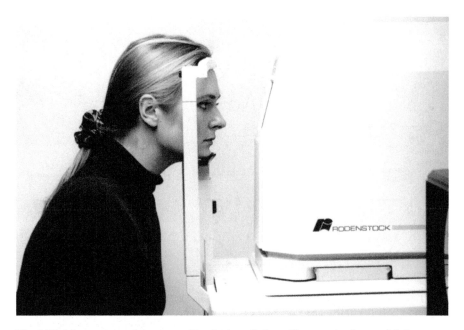

Fig. 1.25   Measurement of the eye position in the roll plane. The scanning laser ophthalmoscope (SLO) can be used to make photographs of the fundus of the eye (examination is also possible with a fundus camera). The rolling of the eye or eye torsion can be measured in degrees on the fundus photographs as the angle between the horizontal and the so-called papillofoveal meridian. The patient sits upright, looks into the SLO, and fixates a dot. (With the SLO, it is not necessary to administer a mydriatic drug; however, this is necessary if the measurement is made with traditional fundus photography.) Both eyes of healthy controls exhibit a slightly excyclotropic position in the roll plane, i.e., counterclockwise rotation of the right eye and a clockwise rotation of the left eye (from the viewpoint of the examiner). The normal range (±2 SDs) is from −1 to 11.5°. Values outside this range are considered pathological (e.g., patients with a peripheral vestibular lesion show an ipsiversive excyclotropia)

- Vestibular Neuritis: The VEMP are actually preserved in two-thirds of the patients. This is due to the sparing of the pars inferior of the vestibular nerve, which supplies the major parts of the saccule and the posterior canal (Rosengren et al. 2010).
- Superior Canal Dehiscence Syndrome (SCDS): The stimulus threshold for inducing cVEMP is typically reduced in most cases (Minor et al. 1998), i.e., a stimulus reaction with elevated amplitude occurs already at low dB values.
- Vestibular Schwannoma: The cVEMP can be absent or reduced.
- Bilateral Vestibulopathy: The cVEMP are absent in only a part of the patients; this should be interpreted as a sign of additional damage of the saccule function (Zingler et al. 2008).

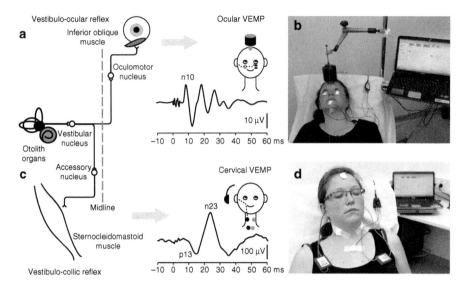

Fig. 1.26 (**a–d**) Vestibular-evoked myogenic potentials (VEMP): ocular VEMP (oVEMP) and cervical VEMP (cVEMP). The VEMP have become an important and clinically relevant examination technique for otolith function. Schematic drawing (**a**) and recording (**b**) of the oVEMP. The stimulation for the oVEMP is usually by vibration or head tapping, preferably with the so-called mini-shaker on the forehead and recording over the inferior oblique muscle while the subject is looking upward. In healthy subjects, one sees a contralateral negative wave (n10) and a positive (p15) wave. This test allows an evaluation of the function of the utricle. The cVEMP (**c**, **d**) allow measurement of the function of the saccule via the vestibulocollic reflex over the vestibular nerves, vestibular nuclei, interneurons, and motor neurons to the neck sternocleidomastoid muscle. The cVEMP are induced by a loud click or burst. Recordings require ca. 50–100 stimulations. The prerequisites for testing the cVEMP are an intact middle-ear function (the hearing function does not have to be retained, since one utilizes the acoustic sensibility of the saccule) and a lifting of head to increase muscle tension. The recording is from a surface EMG of both sternocleidomastoid muscles. Healthy persons show an ipsilateral positive wave (p13) and a negative wave (p23) (Figs. **a** and **c** were kindly provided by Sally Rosengren, Sydney)

- Menière's Disease: The cVEMP are frequently unilateral in the early phase, in the further course bilaterally reduced or absent. This can contribute to the identification of the affected labyrinth.

1.7.4.2   Ocular Vestibular-Evoked Potentials (oVEMP)

The oVEMP are a further development in which the stimulation (best done with a so-called mini-shaker) is induced on the forehead and the potentials are recorded over the oblique inferior muscle while the gaze is directed upward. The signals originate primarily from the utricle and thus are suitable for testing utricle function (Rosengren et al. 2010). It is technically simpler to induce oVEMP than cVEMP, and oVEMP are more and more frequently used. For instance, in vestibular neuritis the amplitude is typically reduced, indicating impaired function of the utricle which is innervated by the superior vestibular nerve typically affected in most patients with this disease.

1.7.5 Pure-Tone Audiogram and Acoustic-Evoked Potentials

ENT physicians test hearing by means of a pure-tone audiogram. In connection with the main symptom of vertigo, audiometry and other tests of the audiological system, e.g., acoustic-evoked potentials or otoacoustic emissions, are of particular importance for diagnosing Menière's disease, vestibular schwannoma, Cogan's syndrome, and other diseases affecting the vestibulocochlear nerve and inner ear.

1.7.6 Posturography and Gait Analysis

Posturography (Fig. 1.27) allows measurement of body sway under different conditions, e.g., with eyes open or closed, or while standing on firm ground or foam rubber. For many years, this method was considered sensitive but not specific. Now with the use of artificial neuronal networks and automatized analysis of the sway patterns under the above-mentioned various conditions, it is possible to decide in many cases whether, for example, a peripheral vestibular deficit, a cerebellar syndrome, an orthostatic tremor, or a phobic postural vertigo is present (Krafczyk et al. 2006; Brandt et al. 2012). A procedure that has proven helpful in the diagnosis and evaluation of treatment effects in various gait disorders is the quantitative gait analysis, for example, of gait variability with the GAITRite, especially in cerebellar disorders (Schniepp et al. 2012a, b).

1.7.7 Additional Laboratory Examinations

To clarify the cause of disorders (differential diagnoses: ischemia, hemorrhage, tumor, inflammation, neurodegenerative disease, malformation, or fracture), additional imaging techniques are necessary, e.g.:

- Cranial magnetic resonance imaging (MRI) with sections of the brainstem, cerebellopontine angle, cerebellum, and labyrinth
- High-resolution computed tomography in particular of the bony labyrinth

If ischemia is suspected, Doppler/duplex sonography is performed, particularly of the vertebral and basilar arteries, and further cardiovascular diagnostics are called for. If a central inflammatory origin is suspected, a spinal tap in addition as well as visual and somatosensory evoked potentials should be performed.

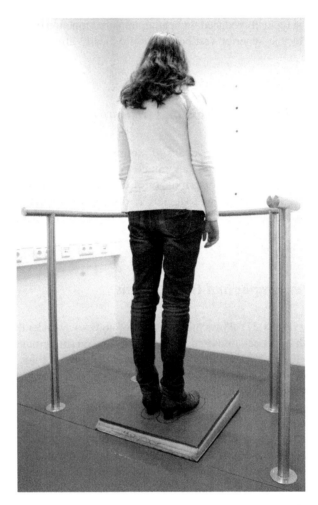

Fig. 1.27 Posturography (here the Kistler platform) allows the examination of control of stance and postural stability under different conditions: eyes open, eyes closed, Romberg and tandem Romberg, or standing on firm ground or on a compliant foam rubber-padded platform. The parameters to be measured are body sway to the right or left, forward or backward, and upward or downward with a subsequent analysis of the so-called sway path values (SP "sway path") and frequency (by a Fourier analysis). The SP is defined as the length of the path described by the center of foot pressure during a given time. Healthy subjects also exhibit body sway as a result of inherent physiological instability. Sway path is increased in patients with a vestibular deficit in particular with the eyes closed. In cerebellar disorders, one finds a typical 3-Hz sway and in orthostatic tremor a 14–16-Hz sway. Nowadays, an automated analysis with an artificial neuronal network allows the differentiation between sensory deficits (namely, vestibular), phobic postural vertigo, cerebellar ataxia, and orthostatic tremor (Krafczyk et al. 2006)

1.7.8   Imaging of the Petrous Bone, the Cerebellopontine Angle, the Brainstem, and Cerebellum with Computed Tomography and Magnetic Resonance Imaging

In general, with high-resolution magnetic resonance imaging (MRI) and computed tomography (CT) of the petrous bone, it is now possible to reliably identify the following peripheral and central vestibular diseases:

- Masses in the cerebellopontine angle, internal auditory canal (e.g., vestibular schwannoma which requires T1 with and without gadolinium and T2 sequences), or middle ear (e.g., cholesteatoma)
- Posttraumatic forms of vertigo due to petrous bone fractures
- "Vestibular pseudoneuritis" due to fascicular lesions of the vestibular nerve at the entry zone of the brainstem (e.g., MS plaques or ischemic lesions)

Imaging is also important for the diagnosis of:

- Inflammatory (e.g., labyrinthitis, Cogan's syndrome), hereditary (e.g., Mondini–Alexander dysplasia), or neoplastic (e.g., meningeosis carcinomatosa) inner-ear diseases
- Vestibular paroxysmia (looking for neurovascular cross-compression of the vestibular nerve)
- Superior canal dehiscence syndrome (looking for a defect of the bone over the superior semicircular canal by high-resolution temporal bone CT and 3-D reconstruction)
- Vestibular neuritis due to herpes zoster virus
- Labyrinthine concussion

Endolymphatic hydrops can be indirectly imaged in cases of Menière's disease by MRI after administering transtympanic gadolinium. So far, BPPV cannot be diagnosed by means of imaging techniques.

1.7.8.1   High-Resolution Computed Tomography of the Petrous Bone

Modern multislice CT machines allow spatially very high-resolution imaging of the petrous bone structures, in particular the bony labyrinth, the facial nerve canal, and the skull base. An examination in the spiral mode of operation (with 1-mm slice thickness, 1-mm table feed, 140 kV, 111 mA, and 0.75 s revolution) yields a local spatial resolution of $0.3 \times 0.3 \times 1$ mm. The data are reconstructed for each side separately. Typically transversal and coronal reconstructions are made; 3-D surface reconstructions are also possible in addition. CT of the petrous bone is indicated when the bone is also to be judged, e.g., to prove presence of fractures, malformations (Mondini–Alexander dysplasia), and in particular the SCDS as well as ossifications of the labyrinth in chronic illnesses (e.g., otosclerosis or Cogan's syndrome) and accompanying bone alterations in benign and malignant growth processes (e.g., cholesteatoma, cholesterol cysts, jugular diverticulitis, vestibular schwannoma, rhabdomyosarcoma, basalioma, or adenocarcinoma).

1.7.8.2   High-Resolution Magnetic Resonance Imaging of the Petrous Bone and the Cerebellopontine Angle

The MRI examination of the petrous bone and the cerebellopontine angle is performed in a circularly polarized head coil. This technique is clearly superior to CT as regards the imaging of non-osseous structures or lesions, e.g., tumors and inflammatory soft-tissue growths, especially in the petrous bone. The numerous anatomical structures confined in a very small space within the petrous bone make high demands on the MRI technology. The examination protocol should include the following (or similar) sequences:

- Transversal proton-weighted and T2-weighted fast spin-echo sequence with a double echo in a 3-mm-thick slice and an interslice distance of less than 0.8 mm for evaluating the brainstem and cerebellum.
- A transversal T1-weighted sequence (e.g., 2-D fast low-angle shot, FLASH) with a 2-mm-thick slice and a spatial resolution of ca. 0.55 mm, before and, if applicable, after intravenous administration of an MRI contrast medium. After the contrast medium is applied, it is advisable to perform a coronal imaging in addition.
- A high-resolution, strongly T2-weighted sequence (e.g., 3-D constructive interference in steady-state, CISS or 3-D FIESTA, fast imaging employing steady-state acquisition) of ca. 0.5-mm spatial resolution and 0.6–0.8-mm slice thickness. This sequence is especially suitable for imaging the cerebral nerves and the fluid-filled inner-ear structures. It is the method of choice for detecting a pathological neurovascular cross-compression. Since it is a 3-D sequence, multiple plane reconstructions can be made in all directions, especially also parallel to the course of each cerebral nerve. By using the maximum intensity projection (MIP) procedure, it is possible to represent the signal-intense structures of the inner ear three-dimensionally and in any orientation.
- If a pathological neurovascular cross-compression is suspected, another complementary examination with MR angiography (e.g., TOF, time of flight) is performed. If the TOF-MRA is performed before and after intravenous administration of contrast medium, it is possible to identify and differentiate contacts with arteries as well as with veins.

1.8   General Principles of Therapy

The treatment of the various forms of vertigo includes drug therapy (Tables 1.10 and 1.11; overviews in Huppert et al. 2011; Strupp et al. 2011b), physical therapy, psychotherapeutic measures, and—nowadays only very seldom—surgery. Before

Table 1.10 Antivertiginous and antiemetic drugs

Drug	Dosage	Action
Anticholinergics		
Scopolamine	Transdermal 1.0 mg/72 h	Muscarine antagonist
Antihistamines		
Dimenhydrinate	Tablet (50 mg) every 4–6 h	Histamine (H_1) antagonist
	Suppository (150 mg) 1–2/day	
Benzodiazepines		
Diazepam	Tablet (5 or 10 mg) every 4–6 h or injected solution of 10 mg i.m.	$GABA_A$ agonist
Clonazepam	Tablet (0.5 mg) every 4–6 h	

treatment begins, the patient should be told that the prognosis is generally good, because many vertigo syndromes take a favorable spontaneous course (e.g., due to improvement of the peripheral vestibular function or as a result of central compensation of the vestibular tonus imbalance) and can be successfully treated.

1.8.1   Drug Therapy

There are only four indications for the use of antivertiginous drugs (Table 1.10) such as antihistamines (e.g., dimenhydrinate) or anticholinergics (e.g., scopolamine), and they are exclusively for the symptomatic treatment of dizziness, nausea, and vomiting:

- In acute peripheral or central vestibular disorders (for a maximum of 3 days)
- To prevent nausea and vomiting during liberatory maneuvers for BPPV
- To prevent motion sickness
- In central positional/positioning vertigo with nausea

None of these pharmaceuticals are suitable for long-term treatment, for example, in cases of chronic central or peripheral vestibular vertigo, cerebellar ataxia, or certain forms of positional vertigo. Once the nausea has ceased, antivertiginous drugs or sedatives should not be administered anymore, because according to animal experiments, they can impair or delay central compensation of a peripheral functional disorder and even lead to drug addiction.

Specifically acting pharmaceuticals are nowadays increasingly being used effectively to treat the causes of other forms of vertigo (overview in Table 1.11). Important examples are:

- Steroids to improve the restitution of peripheral vestibular function in cases of acute vestibular neuritis (Strupp et al. 2004)
- Carbamazepine for vestibular paroxysmia (Brandt and Dieterich 1994; Hufner et al. 2008)
- Betahistine in higher doses and as long-term prophylaxis for Menière's disease (Strupp et al. 2008)
- Beta-receptor blockers and topiramate for the prophylaxis of vestibular migraine

Table 1.11 Drug therapy for different vertigo syndromes and for nystagmus

Therapy	Indication	Drug example and dosage
Drug		
Anticonvulsants	Vestibular paroxysmia (neuro-vascular compression)	Carbamazepine (200–600 mg/day)
	Paroxysmal dysarthrophonia and ataxia in MS	Oxcarbazepine (300–600 mg/day)
	Other central vestibular paroxysmias	
	Myokymia of the superior oblique muscle	
	Vestibular epilepsy	Carbamazepine (800–2,000 mg/day) or other anticonvulsants
	Vestibular migraine	For prophylaxis: Topiramate (50–150 mg/day) Valproic acid (600–1,500 mg/day)
Antivertiginous substances	For symptoms of nausea and vomiting in cases of:	See Table 1.10
	Acute peripheral or central vestibular lesion	
	Central "positional vomiting"	
	Prophylaxis for nausea	
	Vomiting due to liberatory maneuvers in BPPV	
	Prevention of motion sickness	
Beta-receptor blocker	Vestibular migraine	For prophylaxis: Metoprolol retard (50–200 mg/day)
Betahistine	Menière's disease	Betahistine dihydrochloride (72–144 mg/day)
Ototoxic antibiotics	Menière's disease	Gentamicin (10–40 mg) transtym-panally at intervals of 8–12 weeks
	Tumarkin's otolithic crisis (vestibular drop attacks)	
Corticosteroids	Acute vestibular neuritis	Methylprednisolone (100 mg/day, reduce dose every 4th day by 20 mg)
	Acute Cogan's syndrome and other autoimmunological inner-ear diseases	Methylprednisolone (1,000 mg/day i.v., reduce according to course)
Potassium channel blockers	Downbeat nystagmus	4-Aminopyridine (2–3 × 5 mg to 10 mg/day), 4-aminopyridine sustained release (1–2 × 10 mg/day), 3,4-diaminopyridine (3 × 10 mg/day)
	Upbeat nystagmus	
	Episodic ataxia type 2	4-Aminopyridine (2–3 × 5 mg/day), 4-aminopyridine sustained release (1–2 × 10 mg/day)
Selective serotonin reuptake inhibitors	Phobic postural vertigo	Citalopram (10–20 mg/day)

- 4-Aminopyridine and 3,4-diaminopyridine for downbeat and upbeat nystagmus, episodic ataxia type 2, and cerebellar gait disorders (Glasauer et al. 2005; Kalla et al. 2004; Schniepp et al. 2012a; Strupp et al. 2003, 2011a)

1.8.2 Physical Therapy

A specific form of balance training is performed to improve central vestibular compensation in cases of peripheral and central vestibular damage. It entails special exercises for the vestibular, somatosensory, and ocular motor systems in order to promote substitution of the missing vestibular information by other systems and central vestibular compensation. The efficacy of this therapy has been proven in animal and clinical experiments, both for acute lesions (e.g., acute unilateral labyrinthine failure due to vestibular neuritis) and for chronic conditions (e.g., due to vestibular schwannoma) (Hillier and McDonnell 2011) (Table 1.12). If correctly performed, liberatory maneuvers or repositioning exercises used in BPPV lead within a few days to the absence of complaints in more than 95 % of all cases (Hillier and McDonnell 2011).

1.8.3 Psychological/Psychiatric and Behavioral Treatment

Phobic postural vertigo is the second most frequent type of vertigo in our dizziness outpatient unit, and as such, its treatment is of special importance. Treatment

Table 1.12 Physiotherapeutic and operative treatment strategies for vertigo

Treatment strategy	Indications
Physical treatments	
Liberatory/positional maneuver:	Benign paroxysmal positioning vertigo:
According to Semont or Epley	Of the posterior canal
According to Lempert and Tiel-Wilck (barbecue) or Gufoni ("decanting")	Of the horizontal canal
According to Yacovino	Of the anterior canal
Vestibular exercises, balance training, gait training	Improvement of the central vestibular compensation of a vestibular tonus difference (e.g., acute unilateral labyrinthine loss)
	Habituation to prevent motion sickness (physical therapy)
Surgery	
Surgical resection or gamma-knife treatment	Tumors (vestibular schwannoma)
Surgical decompression	Arachnoidal cysts of the posterior cranial fossa
Surgical patching (canal plugging)	External perilymph fistulas
	Superior canal dehiscence syndrome
Labyrinthectomy or transection of the vestibular nerve	Menière's disease (last option)
Neurovascular decompression	Vestibular paroxysmia (last option)

consists mainly of a cognitive behavioral therapy involving desensitization by self-exposure to the precipitating situations. This procedure should also be used in cases of secondary psychological, somatoform, or psychiatric disorders in patients with dizziness. Often a combination with drugs, in particular, selective serotonine reuptake inhibitors (SSRIs), is necessary.

1.8.4 Surgery

If vertigo is caused by a vestibular schwannoma or a cavernoma of the brainstem, surgery or gamma-knife—depending on the location, size, and course—are the treatment options. Otherwise, surgery is necessary only in very rare cases of Menière's disease or vestibular paroxysmia when drug therapy fails. Surgery should also be considered in cases of external perilymph fistulas and the SCDS (Table 1.12). In the other forms of vertigo, surgery is of marginal importance compared to other treatments.

References

Bartl K, Lehnen N, Kohlbecher S, Schneider E. Head impulse testing using video-oculography. Ann N Y Acad Sci. 2009;1164:331–3.

Bisdorff A, von Brevern M, Lempert T, Newman-Toker DE. Classification of vestibular symptoms: towards an international classification of vestibular disorders. J Vestib Res. 2009;19:1–13.

Brandt T, Daroff RB. Physical therapy for benign paroxysmal positional vertigo. Arch Otolaryngol. 1980;106:484–5.

Brandt T, Dieterich M. Vestibular paroxysmia: vascular compression of the eighth nerve? Lancet. 1994;343:798–9.

Brandt T, Strupp M, Novozhilov S, Krafczyk S. Artificial neural network posturography detects the transition of vestibular neuritis to phobic postural vertigo. J Neurol. 2012;259:182–4.

Cnyrim CD, Newman-Toker D, Karch C, Brandt T, Strupp M. Bedside differentiation of vestibular neuritis from central "vestibular pseudoneuritis". J Neurol Neurosurg Psychiatry. 2008;79:458–60.

Davis A, Moorjani P. The epidemiology of hearing and balance disorders. In: Luxon LM, Furman JM, Martini A, Stephens D, editors. Textbook of audiological medicine. London: Dunitz M; 2003. p. 89–99.

Glasauer S, Kalla R, Buttner U, Strupp M, Brandt T. 4-aminopyridine restores visual ocular motor function in upbeat nystagmus. J Neurol Neurosurg Psychiatry. 2005;76:451–3.

Halmagyi GM, Curthoys IS. A clinical sign of canal paresis. Arch Neurol. 1988;45:737–9.

Hillier SL, McDonnell M. Vestibular rehabilitation for unilateral peripheral vestibular dysfunction. Cochrane Database Syst Rev. 2011;2, CD005397.

Hufner K, Barresi D, Glaser M, Linn J, Adrion C, Mansmann U, et al. Vestibular paroxysmia: diagnostic features and medical treatment. Neurology. 2008;71:1006–14.

Huppert D, Strupp M, Muckter H, Brandt T. Which medication do I need to manage dizzy patients? Acta Otolaryngol. 2011;131:228–41.

Kalla R, Glasauer S, Schautzer F, Lehnen N, Büttner U, Strupp M, et al. 4-aminopyridine improves downbeat nystagmus, smooth pursuit, and VOR gain. Neurology. 2004;62:1228–9.

Krafczyk S, Tietze S, Swoboda W, Valkovic P, Brandt T. Artificial neural network: a new diagnostic posturographic tool for disorders of stance. Clin Neurophysiol. 2006;117:1692–8.

Minor LB, Solomon D, Zinreich JS, Zee DS. Sound- and/or pressure-induced vertigo due to bone dehiscence of the superior semicircular canal. Arch Otolaryngol Head Neck Surg. 1998;124: 149–258.

Neuhauser HK. Epidemiology of vertigo. Curr Opin Neurol. 2007;20:40–6.

Newman-Toker DE, Kattah JC, Alvernia JE, Wang DZ. Normal head impulse test differentiates acute cerebellar strokes from vestibular neuritis. Neurology. 2008;70:2378–85.

Rosengren SM, Welgampola MS, Colebatch JG. Vestibular evoked myogenic potentials: past, present and future. Clin Neurophysiol. 2010;121:636–51.

Royl G, Ploner CJ, Mockel M, Leithner C. Neurological chief complaints in an emergency room. Nervenarzt. 2010;81:1226–30.

Schniepp R, Wuehr M, Neuhaeusser M, Benecke AK, Adrion C, Brandt T, ct al. 4-Aminopyridine and cerebellar gait: a retrospective case series. J Neurol. 2012a;259:2491–3.

Schniepp R, Wuehr M, Neuhaeusser M, Kamenova M, Dimitriadis K, Klopstock T, et al. Locomotion speed determines gait variability in cerebellar ataxia and vestibular failure. Mov Disord. 2012b;27:125–31.

Strupp M, Schuler O, Krafczyk S, Jahn K, Schautzer F, Büttner U, et al. Treatment of downbeat nystagmus with 3,4-diaminopyridine: a placebo-controlled study. Neurology. 2003;61: 165–70.

Strupp M, Zingler VC, Arbusow V, Niklas D, Maag KP, Dieterich M, et al. Methylprednisolone, valacyclovir, or the combination for vestibular neuritis. N Engl J Med. 2004;351:354–61.

Strupp M, Hupert D, Frenzel C, Wagner J, Zingler V, Mansmann U, et al. Long-term prophylactic treatment of attacks of vertigo in Meniere's disease – comparison of a high with a low dosage of betahistine in an open trial. Acta Otolaryngol. 2008;128:520–4.

Strupp M, Kalla R, Claassen J, Adrion C, Mansmann U, Klopstock T, et al. A randomized trial of 4-aminopyridine in EA2 and related familial episodic ataxias. Neurology. 2011a;77:269–75.

Strupp M, Thurtell MJ, Shaikh AG, Brandt T, Zee DS, Leigh RJ. Pharmacotherapy of vestibular and ocular motor disorders, including nystagmus. J Neurol. 2011b;258:1207–22.

Zingler VC, Weintz E, Jahn K, Bötzel K, Wagner J, Huppert D, et al. Saccular function less affected than canal function in bilateral vestibulopathy. J Neurol. 2008;255:1332–6.

Zwergal A, Rettinger N, Frenzel C, Frisen L, Brandt T, Strupp M. A bucket of static vestibular function. Neurology. 2009;72:1689–92.

Chapter 2
Peripheral Vestibular Forms of Vertigo

2.1 Introduction and Classification

Three forms of peripheral vestibular disorders, each with its typical symptoms and clinical signs, can be differentiated functionally, anatomically, and pathophysiologically (Table 2.1).

Table 2.1 Three forms of peripheral vestibular disorders

Type of disorder	Main symptoms	Examples and causes
1. Chronic bilateral peripheral vestibular functional deficit	Gait and stance instability that increases in the dark and on unlevel ground (reduced or absent visual or somatosensory information) Oscillopsia during head movements (loss of vestibulo-ocular reflexes) Disorders of spatial memory and navigation	Bilateral vestibulopathy due to: Ototoxic substances (aminoglycosides) Bilateral Menière's disease Meningitis Bilateral acoustic neuroma (neurofibromatosis 2) Hemosiderosis Neurodegenerative with or without additional cerebellar syndrome
2. Acute/subacute unilateral vestibular functional deficit (labyrinth and/or vestibular nerve) with vestibular tonus imbalance	Acute rotatory vertigo (for days or a few weeks) Oscillopsia due to spontaneous nystagmus Tendency to fall in specific direction Nausea	Vestibular neuritis due to reactivation of a latent herpes simplex virus 1 infection (see p.76 and p.115)
3. Inadequate unilateral paroxysmal stimulation or inhibition of the peripheral vestibular system	Attacks with rotatory or postural vertigo depending on cause, with or without triggers, of various duration and with accompanying symptoms	Benign paroxysmal positioning vertigo due to canalolithiasis Menière's disease due to rupture of the endolymphatic membrane Vestibular paroxysmia due to neurovascular compression Perilymph fistula due to changes in pressure

T. Brandt et al., *Vertigo and Dizziness*,
DOI 10.1007/978-0-85729-591-0_2, © Springer-Verlag London 2013

2.2   Benign Paroxysmal Positioning Vertigo

2.2.1   Patient History

The main symptoms of benign paroxysmal positioning vertigo (BPPV) include brief, second-long, sometimes severe attacks of rotatory vertigo with and without nausea. They are caused by rapid changes in head position relative to gravity. Typical triggers include:

- Lying down
- Sitting up in bed
- Rolling over in bed
- Bending over
- Extending the head backward in order to look up or do something above the head.

If BPPV is elicited while the patient is upright, he/she is in danger of falling. Attacks of vertigo are variable: they frequently occur in the morning ("morning vertigo"), after which there often are no effects for hours or days, and are most pronounced during the first change in position after sleep; repeated changes in position cause a transient lessening of the attacks. The complaints are so typical that a diagnosis can often be made solely on the basis of the patient history; occasionally, even the affected ear can be identified ("rotatory vertigo only occurs when lying down on my right side"). The diagnosis of BPPV requires positioning maneuvers that result in a canal-specific positional nystagmus of the posterior, horizontal, or anterior (pc-BPPV > hc-BPPV > ac-BPPV) semicircular canals.

2.2.2   Clinical Features and Course

BPPV is the most common cause of vertigo, not only in the elderly (Table 1.1). Its lifetime prevalence is around 3 % (von Brevern et al. 2007). This condition is characterized by brief attacks of rotatory vertigo and simultaneous positioning rotatory-linear nystagmus toward the forehead and toward the undermost ear. It can be accompanied by nausea. BPPV is elicited by extending the head or positioning the head or body toward the affected ear. Rotatory vertigo and nystagmus occur after such positioning with a short latency of seconds in the form of a crescendo–decrescendo course of 30–60 s. The beating direction of the nystagmus is vertical and rotating in pc-BPPV; it also depends on the direction of gaze and is primarily

- Rotating when gaze is to the undermost ear
- Mostly vertical (to the forehead) during gaze to the uppermost ear

In pc-BPPV, the nystagmus corresponds to an (ampullofugal) excitation of the posterior canal of the undermost ear.

BPPV can appear at any time from childhood to senility, but the idiopathic form is typically a disease of the elderly, peaking in the sixth to seventh decades. More than 95 % of all cases are classified as degenerative or idiopathic (women/men = 2:1), whereas the symptomatic cases (women/men = 1:1) are most frequently caused by head injury (17 %) or vestibular neuritis (15 %) (Karlberg et al. 2000). BPPV also occurs strikingly often in cases of extensive bed rest in connection with other ill-nesses or after operations. About 5 % of the spontaneous cases and 10 % of the trauma cases show a bilateral, generally asymmetrically pronounced BPPV. The right posterior canal is affected about twice as often as the left, which might be con-nected with the fact that more people sleep on their right side (Lopez-Escamez et al. 2002). We found that the history of the disorder until its diagnosis had lasted more than 4 weeks in 50 % of our patients and more than 6 months in 10 %. It is called benign because it generally resolves spontaneously within weeks to months; if not treated, BPPV persists in about 30 % of patients (Imai et al. 2005).

2.2.3 Pathophysiology and Therapeutic Principles

The canalolithiasis hypothesis (Brandt and Steddin 1993; Steddin and Brandt 1996) can explain all symptoms of positional nystagmus. According to this hypothesis, the attacks are induced by otoconia that move freely in the semicircular canal. The movement of the conglomerate causes an ampullofugal or ampullopetal deflection of the cupula depending on the direction of sedimentation and thus leads to a stimu-lation or inhibition of the vestibular hair cells.

This model of the pathomechanism of BPPV can predict the direction, latency, duration, and fatigability of the typical nystagmus, as well as changes in these parameters after other head maneuvers (Fig. 2.1).

2.2.3.1 Latency

Rotatory vertigo and nystagmus appear as soon as the particles in the canal precipi-tate as a result of gravity. This causes a deflection of the cupula, which exceeds the stimulus threshold of the sensory epithelium after 1–5 s.

2.2.3.2 Duration

After the change in position, the particles move toward the lowest point within the canal relative to gravity and precipitate. Depending on their size and composition, this takes about 10 s.

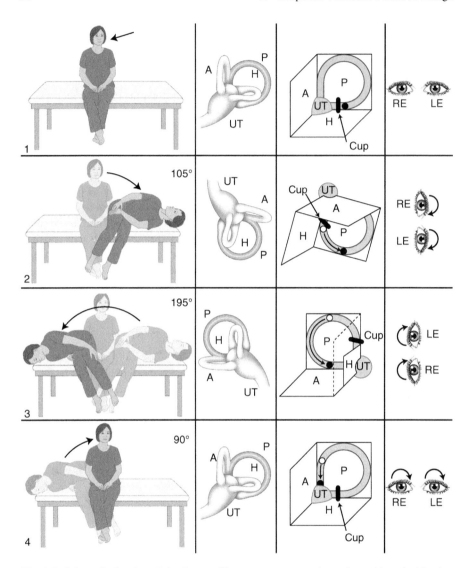

Fig. 2.1 Schematic drawing of the Semont liberatory maneuver of a patient with typical benign paroxysmal positioning vertigo of the left ear. Panels from *left to right*: position of body and head, position of labyrinth in space, position and movement of the clot in the posterior canal (which causes cupula deflection), and the direction of the vertical–torsional nystagmus. The clot is depicted as an *open circle* within the canal; a *black circle* represents the final resting position of the clot. (*1*) In the sitting position, the head is turned horizontally 45° to the unaffected ear. The clot, which is heavier than endolymph, settles at the base of the left posterior semicircular canal. (*2*) The patient is tilted approximately 105° to the left (affected) ear. The change in head position, relative to gravity, causes the clot to gravitate to the lowermost part of the canal and the cupula to deflect downward, inducing BPPV with rotatory nystagmus beating toward the undermost ear. The patient maintains this position for 1 min. (*3*) The patient is turned approximately 195° with the nose down, causing the clot to move toward the exit of the canal. The endolymphatic flow again deflects the cupula such that the nystagmus beats toward the left ear, now uppermost. The patient remains in this position for 1 min. (*4*) The patient is slowly moved into the sitting position; this causes the clot to enter the utricular cavity (adapted from Brandt et al. (1994)). *A, P, H* anterior, posterior, horizontal semicircular canals, *Cup* cupula, *UT* utricular cavity, *RE* right eye, *LE* left eye

2.2.3.3   Course of Attacks

After the positioning, the particles fall away from the curved canal wall. They are accelerated from standstill by the forces of gravity, reach a maximal speed during their fall, and return to standstill at the lowest point in the canal. This explains the temporal crescendo–decrescendo-like course of the attacks; the cupula time constant and the central velocity storage mechanism increase the duration of the nystagmus and vertigo.

2.2.3.4   Direction of Nystagmus

The ampullofugal stimulation of the posterior canal causes compensatory eye movements around the axis of ocular rotation, which is perpendicular to the canal plane, by means of the vestibulo-ocular reflex (VOR). To the physician, this will appear to be a combination of linear (toward the forehead) and rotatory (toward the undermost ear) eye movements.

2.2.3.5   Reversal of Nystagmus

If the direction of the positioning movement is reversed when sitting up, the particles move in the opposite direction. Now the cupula is deflected in the opposite (ampullopetal) direction. This results in a reversal of both the rotatory vertigo and the direction of nystagmus due to inhibition of the vestibular hair cells.

2.2.3.6   Fatigability

The particles that form a plug or clump are loosely held together. They fall apart more and more during changes in the head position. Small particles cannot cause as much suction or pressure on the cupula independently of each other, as does a single clump, whose volume almost fills the canal. If the patient holds his head still for several hours (e.g., during sleep), the particles, which had fallen apart before, coalesce into a clump in the lowest place within the canal and again induce vertigo when the head position is changed.

2.2.3.7   Liberatory Maneuver

The efficacy of positioning (liberatory) maneuvers of the head can only be explained by the canalolithiasis hypothesis, i.e., the clot moves freely within the canal. By quickly moving the patient's head to the opposite side, the plug is washed out of the canal and then can no longer cause any positioning vertigo

(Brandt and Steddin 1993; Brandt et al. 1994). Brandt and Daroff in 1980 first devised an effective exercise program, which, by means of the simple physical measure of head positioning, loosens the heavy degenerative otolithic material and distributes it into other areas of the labyrinth, where it comes to rest and no longer impairs canal function. This effective method has been modified; we nowadays recommend that the patient's position—according to the modified "liberatory maneuver" of Semont et al. (1988)—be changed from the inducing position by a tilt of 180° to the opposite side (Fig. 2.1). In 1992, Epley proposed another liberatory maneuver that involved turning the patient from a supine position into a head-hanging position (Fig. 2.2). Evidence-based reviews conclude that all maneuvers are effective (Fife et al. 2008) and can be explained by the mechanism of canalolithiasis (Brandt et al. 1994; Strupp et al. 2007). The success rate of the Semont as well as the Epley maneuver is around 90 % (meta-analyses).

2.2.4 Pragmatic Therapy

2.2.4.1 Physical Liberatory Maneuvers

When correctly performed, the physical liberatory maneuvers according to Semont (Semont et al. 1988) or Epley's repositioning maneuver (Epley 1992) are successful in almost all patients (Strupp et al. 2007). We recommend Semont's liberatory maneuver depicted in Fig. 2.1 as the therapy of first choice. If it fails despite correct performance, the Epley maneuver (Fig. 2.2) can be carried out. The Brandt–Daroff maneuver (Fig. 2.3) can be used in special cases, for example, in cases of cupulolithiasis of the horizontal canal in order to transform it into a canalolithiasis (see below).

Fig. 2.2 Schematic drawing of modified Epley liberatory maneuver. Patient characteristics and abbreviations are as in Fig. 2.1. (*1*) In the sitting position, the head is turned horizontally 45° to the affected (*left*) ear. (*2*) The patient is tilted approximately 105° backward into a slightly head-hanging position, causing the clot to move in the canal, deflecting the cupula downward, and inducing the paroxysmal positioning vertigo. The patient remains in this position for 1 min. (*3a*) The head is turned 90° to the unaffected ear, now undermost, and (*3b*) the head and trunk continue turning another 90° to the right, causing the clot to move toward the exit of the canal. The patient remains in this position for 1 min. The positioning nystagmus beating toward the affected (*uppermost*) ear in positions 3a and 3b indicates effective therapy. (*4*) The patient is moved into the sitting position (adapted from Brandt et al. (1994))

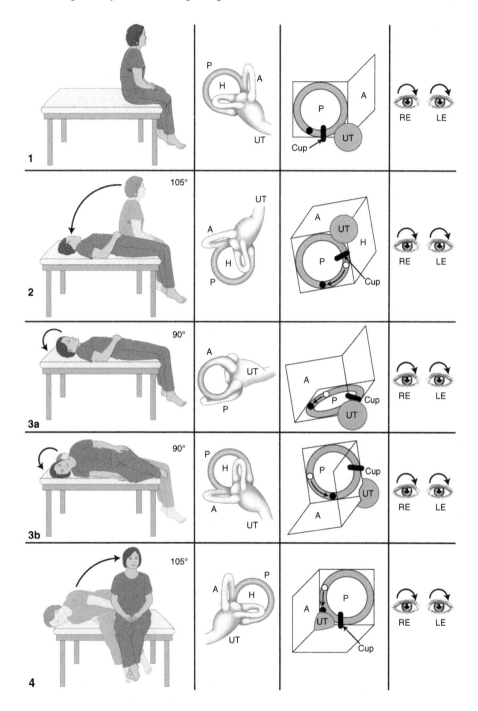

Fig. 2.3 Schematic drawing of a positioning maneuver of a patient with benign paroxysmal positioning vertigo (adapted from Brandt and Daroff 1980). *Above* are shown the initial sitting position and the side positioning with somewhat oblique head position; each position should be held for 20–30 s for physical therapy. These positionings are performed serially several times a day. *Below*: a schematic drawing of canalolithiasis

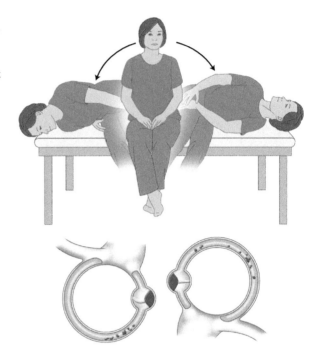

2.2.4.2 Semont Maneuver

According to the liberatory maneuver developed by Semont—even before the mechanism of canalolithiasis was known—the patient's head is first rotated by 45° to the side of the healthy labyrinth in order to bring the posterior canal into the plane of the positioning maneuver (Semont et al. 1988). Then the patient is turned 90° to the side of the affected labyrinth; he/she holds this position for about 1 min. Afterward comes the so-called great toss: the patient is turned by 180° to the side of the *unaffected* labyrinth, where he/she again has to remain lying for at least 1 min. Positional nystagmus to the uppermost ear (Fig. 2.1, panel 3) indicates that the plug has left the canal, i.e., the therapy is successful. Conversely, positional nystagmus to the lowermost healthy ear indicates that the liberatory maneuver failed and the procedure must be repeated (Fig. 2.4). Finally, the patient sits up. This maneuver should be repeated three times each: in the morning, afternoon, and evening until the patient is symptom-free. The efficacy of the Semont maneuver appears to be somewhat less than that of the Epley maneuver (see below). There has been a randomized study with an untreated control group: after one or multiple treatments 94 % of the patients as opposed to only 36 % of the controls were symptom-free (Salvinelli et al. 2003). In another double-blind sham-controlled study, 1 h after one Semont maneuver 79 % and 24 h later 87 % were symptom-free compared to none within the sham group (Mandala et al. 2012). According to older retrospective case series, the success rate of the Semont maneuver is around 50–70 % after one treatment and over

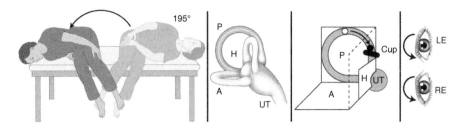

Fig. 2.4 Schematic drawing of an ineffective liberatory maneuver (compare with Fig. 2.1, panel 3). After the patient with left-sided benign paroxysmal positioning vertigo is tilted from the symptomatic position to the right, the particles do not leave the canal but sediment once again ampullopetally onto the cupula. This causes an ampullopetal cupula deflection with positioning nystagmus, which in this position beats downward toward the unaffected right ear. This indicates that the liberatory maneuver has failed and must be repeated (adapted from Brandt et al. (1994))

90–98 % after several treatments (Semont et al. 1988; Serafini et al. 1996; Steenerson and Cronin 1996; Coppo et al. 1996; Levrat et al. 2003).

2.2.4.3   Epley Maneuver

Epley's repositioning maneuver requires that the supine patient's head and trunk be rotated after being tilted backward into a slightly head-hanging position (Epley 1992) (Fig. 2.2). Its efficacy has been proven in the meantime by five controlled, randomized studies and meta-analyses (Lynn et al. 1995; Froehling et al. 2000; Yimtae et al. 2003; Cohen and Kimball 2004; von Brevern et al. 2006b; Strupp et al. 2007). Another meta-analysis has shown that patients in the first follow-ups were 4.6-times more symptom-free than untreated patients (Woodworth et al. 2004). After the first positioning maneuver, about 40–60 % of the patients are symptom-free and after the third maneuver, about 94–98 % (Steenerson and Cronin 1996). For the Epley maneuver to be successful, the following details must be kept in mind:

1. The transition from one position to the next is performed quickly but not abruptly.
2. Patients with restricted movement of the neck are treated either on an examination couch with lowered headrest or alternatively with the Semont maneuver.
3. In cases of pronounced fear or nausea, we recommend administering premedication with dimenhydrinate or other antivertiginous drugs about 30 min before beginning the exercises.
4. The success rate is improved by repeating the maneuver two to three times in one session (Gordon and Gadoth 2004).
5. The success rate is not improved by Epley's original suggestion to vibrate the mastoid bone during the maneuver (Hain et al. 2000; Macias et al. 2004; Ruckenstein and Shepard 2007).
6. The recommendation to remain upright for 48 h after a successful treatment to avoid early recurrences has proved unnecessary (Marciano and Marcelli 2000; Roberts et al. 2005). The same is true for the Semont maneuver (Massoud and Ireland 1996).

The occurrence of an orthotropic nystagmus (the so-called liberatory nystagmus) in the second step of the Epley maneuver indicates that the treatment will be successful (Brandt and Steddin 1993; Oh et al. 2007).

A direct comparison of the Semont and Epley maneuvers found no differences (Cohen and Jerabek 1999; Herdman and Tusa 1996; Massoud and Ireland 1996; Soto-Varela et al. 2001; Steenerson and Cronin 1996). The choice of the maneuver to be used should depend on which maneuver the therapist has the most experience with or if there are any individual contraindications. Very obese patients are easier to treat with the Epley method, while the Semont maneuver or the Brandt–Daroff maneuver (Fig. 2.3) is more suitable for patients with shoulder–neck problems.

Transient nausea can occur as an accompanying effect, above all during repeated positionings within one sitting (prophylaxis with, e.g., 100 mg dimenhydrinate or another antivertiginous substance is indicated). About 20–40 % of the successfully treated patients experience 1–2 weeks of light-headedness or postural vertigo with gait instability (most likely otolith vertigo) due to the partial repositioning of the otoconia toward the utricle (von Brevern et al. 2006a). Occasionally, a positional vertigo of the posterior vertical canal converts into the horizontal or anterior canal variants due to the treatment (Herdman and Tusa 1996).

2.2.4.4 Self-Treatment

The Epley and Semont maneuvers can be successfully applied by the patient him/herself (Radtke et al. 2004). The treatment is performed three times in the morning, three times at noon and three times at night until no symptoms are present. A thorough guidance by demonstration and pictures is necessary. The success rates (50–90 % after 1 week) are not as high as when a physician performs the maneuver. Thus, the self-therapy can be used in a complementary way, for example, in patients with remaining complaints or frequent recurrences. Patients who fail to get along with these maneuvers can perform the easier Brandt–Daroff exercises, which were the first effective physical therapy of BPPV. However, as a rule it takes longer until the patient is symptom-free (Radtke et al. 1999).

2.2.4.5 Recurrences After Successful Liberatory Maneuvers

According to follow-up observations made over an average of 10 years, the recurrence rate in treated patients totals about 50 %. Of these patients, 80 % have recurrences in the first year independently of the type of liberatory maneuver applied (Brandt et al. 2006). Women have a rate of 58 % and thus are more often affected than men who have a rate of 39 %. The recurrence rate is less in the seventh decade than in the sixth decade. Treatment in such cases is an appropriate liberatory maneuver of the affected canal.

2.2.4.6   Surgery

Surgery is very seldom necessary, and if it is, then only in cases refractive to correct liberatory maneuvers. In our collective of several thousands of patients with BPPV, this was only once the case. Then an operative sectioning of the posterior canal nerve can be performed. Selective neurectomy is difficult and there is a risk of hearing loss. Neurectomy has now been replaced by operative closure (plugging) of the posterior canal. This is a safer and effective measure, which, however, in our opinion is performed too frequently in certain centers, i.e., before all the possibilities of simple, effective physical therapy are exhausted.

2.2.4.7   Additional Medication

Since first studies have demonstrated an association of osteopenia/osteoporosis with idiopathic BPPV (Jeong et al. 2009), serum vitamin D levels should be measured especially in older women. Patients with idiopathic BPPV showed a higher prevalence of decreased serum vitamin D than age- and gender-matched controls (Jeong et al. 2013). Thus, decreased serum vitamin D may be a risk factor for BPPV and can probably explain the predominance of women (2:1) with degenerative or idiopathic type of BPPV.

2.2.4.8   Ineffective Measures

Because of the pathomechanism of BPPV, neither are antivertiginous substances causally possible nor are drugs sufficiently effective against the symptoms in the long term. The only exceptions are sensitive patients who develop severe nausea after a single maneuver. In this case, the administration of, for example, dimenhydrinate (100 mg) half an hour before performing the liberatory maneuvers can make therapy easier.

2.2.5   Benign Paroxysmal Positional Vertigo of the Horizontal Canal (hc-BPPV)

BPPV of the horizontal canal (McClure 1985) is less frequent than pc-BPPV but is still diagnosed too seldom. Its key features differ from those of pc-BPPV:

- It can be induced by turning the head along the longitudinal axis of the supine body (either to the right or to the left) (Fig. 2.5). In a canalolithiasis of the horizontal canal this results in an ampullopetal deflection of the cupula when the head is turned to the side of the affected ear with more severe vertigo and nystagmus.

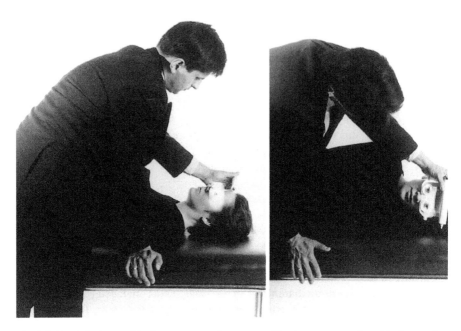

Fig. 2.5 Precipitating positioning maneuvers for suspected benign paroxysmal positioning vertigo of the horizontal semicircular canal (hc-BPPV) by turning the head (to the right as well as to the left) along the longitudinal axis of the body while the subject is supine. When the head is turned to the side of the affected ear, there is an ampullopetal deflection of the cupula (and thus stimulation of the vestibular hair cells) in canalolithiasis. This causes a more severe vertigo and nystagmus than when turned to the unaffected ear

- The beating direction of nystagmus corresponds to the stimulation or inhibition of the horizontal canal, i.e., in canalolithiasis it beats linearly and horizontally to the undermost ear.
- Repeated positioning maneuvers cause hardly any fatigue of the positional nystagmus.
- The duration of the attacks and the nystagmus is longer because of the horizontal canal's so-called central storage mechanism of velocity. Positional nystagmus frequently shows a reversal of direction during the attacks; this corresponds to postrotatory nystagmus (the so-called P I and P II).

The typical case of hc-BPPV can also be explained by canalolithiasis (Strupp et al. 1995), although it has occasionally been observed that the mechanism switches from canalolithiasis to cupulolithiasis (Steddin and Brandt 1996). In the rare form of hc-BPPV due to cupulolithiasis (characterized by nystagmus beating horizontally to the uppermost ear with a lower intensity on the affected side), the "zero point" of positional nystagmus (beyond which direction changes) can be determined by turning the patient's head 10–20° around the longitudinal axis while in the supine position; this is possible because the cupula of the ipsilateral horizontal canal is then parallel to the gravity vector (Bisdorff and Debatisse 2001). In this way, one can also determine which side is affected by hc-BPPV.

We assume that persistent hc-BPPV occurs when there is a certain narrowness of the canal and the congealed clump cannot leave the canal (which narrows toward its exit in an ampullofugal direction) because of its size. Otherwise, it could be assumed that the particles would independently and inevitably leave the canal with every accidental rotation around the longitudinal axis of the body (e.g., in bed). The striking feature of hc-BPPV, i.e., it does not fatigue, agrees with this assumption, as does the general experience that hc-BPPV is difficult to treat with single positioning maneuvers.

2.2.5.1 Therapy for Horizontal BPPV

Therapy involves rotations around the patient's longitudinal axis while recumbent. In essence, this is an altered version of the Epley maneuver. For canalolithiasis, the supine patient is rotated in three 90° steps around the longitudinal axis toward the healthy ear. The patient holds each position for 30 s (Lempert and Tiel-Wilck 1996). An effective alternative is to assume a lateral recumbent position on the side of the healthy ear for 12 h (Vannucchi et al. 2000). A comparative study showed success rates of 70 % for both maneuvers after one application as opposed to 30 % in the untreated controls (Nuti et al. 1998). The combination of both maneuvers (the modified Epley maneuver followed by a lateral recumbent position) is successful in about 90 % of the patients (Casani et al. 2002). The success rate can reach 100 % after 3 rotations along the longitudinal axis (Steenerson et al. 2005). Alternatively one can perform the so-called Gufoni maneuver (Gufoni et al. 1998) (Fig. 2.6), with which patients with either a canalolithiasis or a cupulolithiasis can be successfully treated (Kim et al. 2012a, b). The advantage of this maneuver is that one must not determine which form of an hc-BPPV is present. While in a sitting position, the patient is simply laid down on the side exhibiting less nystagmus. Afterward, the head is turned 45° downward ("decanting") and then sit up (Gufoni et al. 1998; Casani et al. 2002; Asprella 2005).

2.2.6 BPPV of the Anterior Canal (ac-BPPV)

The main symptoms of ac-BPPV correspond to those of pc-BPPV. The clinical examination during the diagnostic positioning maneuvers finds, however, a vertical nystagmus that beats downward and has torsional components (Imai et al. 2006). The relative frequency of ac-BPPV is low: a study reported that it occurred in 2.2 % of 577 patients with BPPV (Yacovino et al. 2009). The same group devised a new and simple maneuver to treat ac-BPPV. From a head-hanging position, the patient must bow his head 30° toward the chest and after 1 min sit up. This study reported a success rate of 85 % after one single maneuver (Yacovino et al. 2009). This high success rate does not correspond to our experience. Further studies should verify their findings.

Fig. 2.6 Gufoni maneuver for treating horizontal semicircular canal BPPV (adapted from Casani et al. (2002), which is modified from Gufoni et al. (1998)). The maneuver is very easy, because one places the patient simply on the side with less nystagmus (regardless of whether it is a geotropic or apogeotropic variant) and then the patient (**a–c**) and then sits up

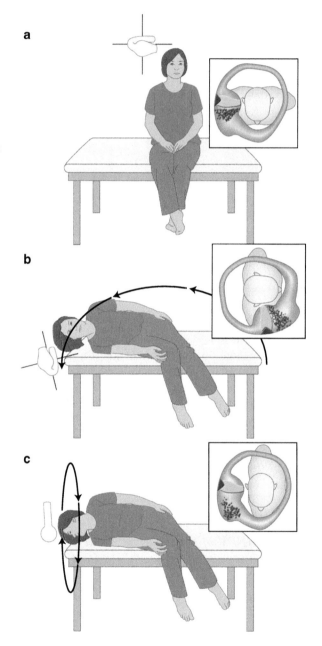

2.2.7   *Differential Diagnosis and Clinical Problems*

The diagnosis of BPPV can in most cases be made on the basis of a typical patient history (brief rotatory vertigo when turning over or sitting up/lying down in bed) and the clinical findings. Especially in cases of therapy-refractory rotatory vertigo (despite correct positioning exercises), the following syndromes should be considered along with unilateral BPPV in the differential diagnosis:

- Central positional nystagmus (infrequent; see below)
- Bilateral BPPV, particularly posttraumatic (ca. 10 %)
- Hc-BPPV (too rarely diagnosed; see above)
- Vestibular paroxysmia (see Sect. 2.5)
- Central infratentorial lesions that mimic BPPV (very rare).

2.2.8 Central Positional Vertigo/Nystagmus

Central positional vertigo and central positional nystagmus are caused by infratentorial lesions that affect connections between the vestibular nuclei in the medulla oblongata and cerebellar structures close to the midline (mainly nodulus and vermis). It is important to distinguish between peripheral and central vestibular disorders, as the latter require further laboratory diagnostics. Four characteristic forms of central positional vertigo/nystagmus can be distinguished, although the symptoms overlap and combinations occur:

- Central downbeat nystagmus, mainly in head-hanging position (with or without accompanying vertigo), typically with lesions of the nodulus
- Central positional nystagmus (without vertigo)
- Central paroxysmal positional vertigo with nystagmus, typically with nodulus lesions
- "Central positioning vomiting".

These central vestibular disorders occur much more seldom than the typical BPPV. However, it can be difficult to distinguish peripheral and central function disorders in the individual patient (Table 2.2). The following clinical rules are important for diagnosing a central positional vertigo/nystagmus (Büttner et al. 1999):

- Persisting positional nystagmus (slow-phase velocity >5°/s) without associated vertigo.
- Positioning-induced vomiting after single head movements without any substantial vertigo or nystagmus.
- Positional/positioning vertigo with nystagmus of purely torsional or vertical character (downbeat or upbeat directions); a purely horizontal direction of nystagmus is typical for hc-BPPV.
- Positional/positioning nystagmus that does not correspond to the plane of the semicircular canal stimulated or inhibited by the head positioning (e.g., torsional nystagmus after stimulation of the horizontal canal).

In clinical practice, the latter seems to be the most important feature by which a central positional nystagmus can be identified.

According to rules common in the past, positional nystagmus beating toward the uppermost ear or lasting longer than 1 min indicated a central pathology; this is no longer considered a reliable differentiating feature, as both occur with the cupulolithiasis variant of BPPV.

Table 2.2 Clinical features differentiating a benign peripheral paroxysmal positioning vertigo (BPPV) from a central positional vertigo or nystagmus (CPV) (Büttner et al. 1999)

Features	BPPV	CPV
Latency following precipitating positioning maneuvers	1–15 s (shorter in hc-BPPV)	No latency or 1–5 s
Vertigo	Typical	Typical
Duration of attack	5–40 s (longer in hc-BPPV and in rare cupulolithiasis)	5–>60 s
Direction of nystagmus	Torsional–vertical with head positioning in the plane of the posterior (pc-BPPV) or the anterior (ac-BPPV) canal, horizontal with head positioning in the plane of the horizontal (hc-BPPV) canal	Purely vertical or torsional, combined torsional/linear, direction of nystagmus does not correspond with the plane of the canal stimulated or inhibited by the head movement
Course of vertigo and nystagmus in the attack	Crescendo–decrescendo (with typical canalolithiasis)	Crescendo–decrescendo is possible
Nausea and vomiting	Rare with single head-positioning maneuvers (if so, then associated with intense positioning nystagmus), frequent with repeated maneuvers	Frequently with single head-positioning maneuvers (not necessarily associated with intense nystagmus)
Natural course	Spontaneous recovery within days to months in 70–80 %	Dependent on etiology, spontaneous recovery within weeks in most cases
Associated neurological signs and symptoms	None (in idiopathic BPPV)	Frequent cerebellar and ocular motor signs such as ataxia, saccadic pursuit, gaze-evoked nystagmus, downbeat nystagmus, impaired fixation suppression of the VOR
Brain imaging	Normal	Lesions dorsolateral from the fourth ventricle and/or of the nodulus or dorsal vermis (tumor, hemorrhages, infarctions, or multiple sclerosis plaques)
		Less specific lesions (cerebellar degeneration, paraneoplastic syndromes, encephalopathy, intoxication)

2.3   Vestibular Neuritis (Acute Partial Unilateral Vestibular Deficit)

2.3.1   Patient History

The main symptoms of an acute unilateral vestibular deficit are a sustained violent rotatory vertigo with illusory movements of the surroundings (oscillopsia), gait and postural imbalance with a tendency to fall, as well as nausea and vomiting. All of these symptoms have an acute or subacute onset and last for a few days or weeks. As the complaints of the patients are exacerbated by any movements of the head, they intuitively seek peace and quiet. Acute hearing disorders, tinnitus, or other neurological deficits do not belong to the clinical picture of the illness. The patient should be explicitly asked about such symptoms. There are no typical antecedent signs or triggers, except for occasional spells of vertigo a few days before in some patients.

2.3.2   Clinical Features and Course

The clinical syndrome of acute vestibular neuritis is characterized by (Fig. 2.7):

- Persistent rotatory vertigo with oscillopsia and pathological tilting of the subjective visual vertical to the side of the affected labyrinth.
- Horizontal–rotatory peripheral vestibular spontaneous nystagmus (to the nonaffected side); generally it can be suppressed by visual fixation (for this reason, Frenzel's goggles are obligatory for the examination). The nystagmus increases while looking in the direction of the fast phase of the nystagmus.
- Gait deviation and tendency to fall (to the affected side).
- Nausea and vomiting.
- Unilateral functional deficit of the horizontal canal, which can be detected by the head-impulse test according to Halmagyi–Curthoys (clinical examination of the vestibulo-ocular reflex (VOR)) and caloric irrigation.

The diagnosis of vestibular neuritis is one of exclusion. Clinical findings that argue against a diagnosis of vestibular neuritis are the following:

- Vertical divergence (skew deviation, one eye is higher than the other) as a component of the ocular tilt reaction (Cnyrim et al. 2008; Kattah et al. 2009) or central ocular motor signs
- A nonpathological Halmagyi–Curthoys head-impulse test (Newman-Toker et al. 2008)

Fig. 2.7 Symptoms and clinical signs of an acute unilateral labyrinthine deficit. Peripheral vestibular spontaneous nystagmus (quick phase) and rotatory vertigo to the unaffected side occur, accompanied by a tendency to fall, ocular torsion, and deviation of the subjective visual vertical and the subjective straight ahead to the affected side

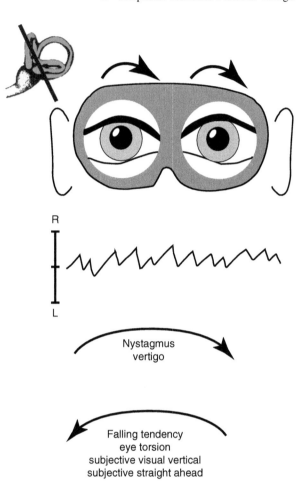

- Gaze-evoked nystagmus in the opposite direction of the fast phase of the spontaneous nystagmus
- Saccadic smooth pursuit
- Central fixation nystagmus, which is typically not suppressed by visual fixation
- Acute hearing disorders or acute tinnitus
- Other deficits involving the cranial nerves, brainstem signs like facial palsy or perioral paresthesia, sensory deficits, headaches, or phono- or photophobia

Vestibular neuritis has an incidence of 3.5 per 100,000 persons (Sekitani et al. 1993). Thus, after BPPV and Menière's disease, it is the third most frequent cause of peripheral vestibular vertigo and accounts for ca. 8 % of the diagnoses made in a specialized neurological outpatient clinic for vertigo. The disease occurs most frequently in adults between 30 and 60 years of age. Short attacks of rotatory vertigo occasionally precede the onset of manifest loss of function by a few days (Lee et al. 2009).

The first phase of manifest loss of function is generally characterized by a severe vertigo, dizziness, and tendency to fall. The complaints are joined by a feeling of illness, nausea, and vomiting. The complaints resolve slowly over 1–2 weeks. As a rule, the patient is generally symptom-free within 3–5 weeks when at rest, i.e., under static conditions. Recovery is the result of a combination of the following:

- Central compensation of the peripheral vestibular tonus imbalance
- Restoration of peripheral vestibular function (generally incomplete)
- Substitution of the functional loss by the contralateral unaffected vestibular system as well as by somatosensory (neck proprioception) and visual input.

In the course of the illness, the peripheral vestibular function does not spontaneously recover in most patients (Brandt et al. 2010). A study with 60 patients showed that after 1 month 90 % and after 6 months 80 % of the patients still had a relevant deficit of peripheral vestibular function. In only 42 % did a normalization occur in the further course (Okinaka et al. 1993). Even in cases in which the peripheral deficit is complete, all "static" symptoms (without head movement) resolve, such as spontaneous nystagmus, vertigo, and a tendency to fall. The remaining deficit, however, is still manifest in the form of a "dynamic" dysfunction: retinal slip of images of the visual scene with oscillopsia during rapid, high-frequency head movements and walking and running because of the insufficiency of the VOR (Halmagyi and Curthoys 1988). Even if the caloric test normalizes in these patients, the head-impulse test on the affected side is pathological in 30 % (Schmid-Priscoveanu et al. 2001). The long-term recurrence rate of vestibular neuritis is between 2 and 11 % (Huppert et al. 2006; Kim et al. 2011a).

2.3.3 Pathophysiology, Etiology, and Therapeutic Principles

Rotatory vertigo and rotating spontaneous nystagmus toward the healthy side are caused by an imbalance of the vestibular tonus between the intact and the disturbed labyrinth. This difference in tonus is due to the fact that the vestibular nerve is active even without head movements: the action potential frequency at rest lies around 100 Hz. The dynamic deficit of the VOR can be proven by a rapid head-impulse test (Halmagyi and Curthoys 1988) when the head is turned to the side of the affected vestibular nerve. The tendency to fall to the side of the lesion might be due to an overcompensation of the tonus imbalance by the vestibulospinal stance reflexes.

Evidently vestibular neuritis tends to affect the superior portion of the vestibular nerves, which supplies the horizontal and anterior canals as well as the utricle and parts of the saccule. The causes are probably the longer and narrower bony canal, through which the superior part passes (Gianoli et al. 2005), and the double supply by the inferior part (Fig. 2.8) (Arbusow et al. 2003). Thus, functionally vestibular neuritis is not equivalent to a total vestibular deficit. This was suspected due to the co-occurrence of vestibular neuritis and BPPV in the same ear (Büchele and Brandt 1988) and later confirmed with three-dimensional (3-D) analysis of the canal function (Fetter and Dichgans 1996). On the basis of 3-D VOR measurements, the rarer subtype of inferior vestibular neuritis (accounting for about less than 10 % of all patients with

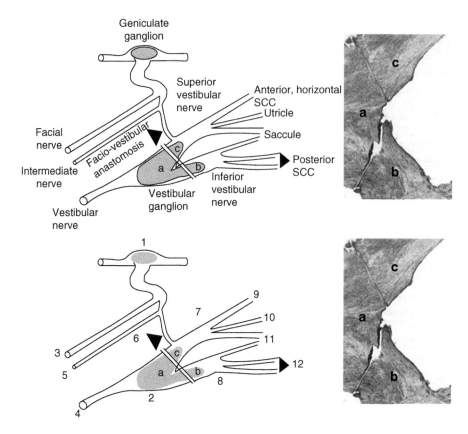

Fig. 2.8 *Left*: schematic drawing of the vestibular and facial nerves, the faciovestibular anastomosis, the geniculate ganglion, and different sections of the vestibular ganglion (*a* stem, *b* inferior portion, *c* superior portion). *Right*: longitudinal cross-section of a human vestibular ganglion, in which the individual portions are separated. The presence of herpes simplex virus-1 DNA in ca. 60 % of all human vestibular ganglia was confirmed by polymerase chain reaction. Moreover, the double innervation of the posterior canal, which may lead to the preservation of its function during vestibular neuritis, is visible (Reproduced with permission from Arbusow et al. (1999)). *1* ganglion geniculi, *2* vestibular ganglion, *3* facial nerve, *4* vestibular nerve, *5* intermediate nerve, *6* faciovestibular anastomoses, *7* superior vestibular nerve, *8* inferior vestibular nerve, *9* anterior, horizontal semicircular canals, *10* utricle, *11* saccule, *12* posterior semicircular canal

vestibular neuritis) has been examined in detail with eye movement vector analysis and vestibular-evoked myogenic potentials (Kim and Kim 2012).

The viral genesis of vestibular neuritis—on the analogy of "idiopathic facial paresis" and several forms of sudden deafness—is probable but not yet confirmed (Baloh 2003; Baloh et al. 1996; Gacek and Gacek 2002; Nadol 1995; Schuknecht and Kitamura 1981). This is supported by autopsy studies (which have shown inflammatory degeneration of the vestibular nerves (Schuknecht 1993)) and by proof of the presence of herpes simplex virus type 1 DNA as well as the latency-associated transcript in the vestibular ganglia (Arbusow et al. 1999, 2000, 2003; Theil et al. 2001, 2002) (Fig. 2.8). The major damage to the nerve is probably a result of the pressure within the bony canal.

2.3.3.1 Therapeutic Principles

The following therapeutic principles are derived from the above-mentioned pathophysiology and etiology.

Symptomatic Therapy for Nausea and Vomiting

Antivertiginous drugs can be administered. They should only be given during the first days and only in cases of severe nausea and vomiting, as they act as sedatives and may delay central compensation of the peripheral vestibular deficit (Dutia 2010).

Causal Therapy

Studies in the 1990s indicated that glucocorticoids can improve the course of "acute vertigo" (Ariyasu et al. 1990; Ohbayashi et al. 1993). A prospective, randomized, placebo-controlled study in 141 patients showed that monotherapy with methylprednisolone significantly improved the peripheral vestibular function of patients with vestibular neuritis (Strupp et al. 2004). Valacyclovir had no influence on the course of the disease, neither as monotherapy nor in combination with methylprednisolone. This proves that corticosteroids are an effective form of treatment for acute vestibular neuritis. These findings are supported by both a meta-analysis (Goudakos et al. 2010) and another study (Karlberg and Magnusson 2011). However, a Cochrane analysis still makes no treatment recommendation for corticosteroids, and the effects on life quality have still not been investigated sufficiently (Fishman et al. 2011).

Improvement of Central Vestibular Compensation

So far, the most important principle of therapy is to promote central compensation by means of physical therapy. This so-called central compensation is not a uniform process. It involves various neural and structural mechanisms that operate in different locations (vestibulospinal or vestibulo-ocular structures) within different time courses, have various limited possibilities, and cause incomplete results, especially as regards head oscillations at high frequencies (Brandt et al. 1997). The central counter-regulation (compensation) of a unilateral labyrinthine lesion is enhanced and accelerated if movement stimuli trigger inadequate and incongruent afferent signals that provoke a sensory mismatch. Vestibular exercises, first recommended by Cawthorne (1944), and later modified according to current knowledge of vestibular function (Hamann 1988; Brandt 1999; Strupp et al. 1998; Herdman 2007), include the following:

- Voluntary eye movements and fixation to improve impaired gaze stabilization
- Active head movements to recalibrate the VOR
- Balance training, goal-directed movements, and gait exercises to improve the vestibulospinal regulation of posture and goal-directed motion.

Animal experiments have proven the efficacy of exercises to promote central compensation of spontaneous nystagmus and to counteract the tendency to fall after

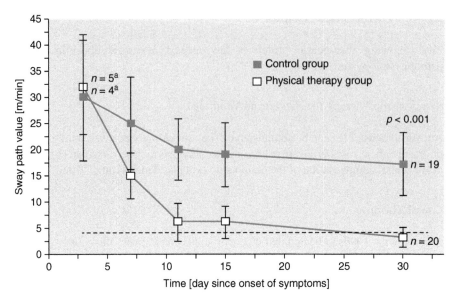

Fig. 2.9 Time course of the changes in total sway path (SP) values for a patient group and a control group, both after acute vestibular neuritis without recovery of the labyrinthine function. Whereas the initial values for SP (m/min, mean $\pm$ SD), measured with eyes closed and standing on a compliant foam rubber-padded posturography platform, were not significantly different in the two groups, the SP values in the therapy group normalized significantly faster in the course of the study. On day 30 (statistical endpoint), there was a significant difference between the two groups (analysis of variance, $p < 0.001$). Thus, balance training improves the vestibulospinal compensation of an acute unilateral peripheral vestibular deficit. The *dotted line* indicates the normal range. [a]During the first days after onset of the illness, some of the patients had such pronounced disturbances of postural control that they were unable to stand on the platform for the amount of time required to perform the measurements (>10 s) without falling (reproduced with permission from Strupp et al. (1998))

unilateral labyrinthine lesions. A prospective, randomized controlled study demonstrated that intensive physiotherapy significantly improved vestibulospinal compensation in patients with acute vestibular neuritis (Strupp et al. 1998) (Fig. 2.9). These findings are supported by a Cochrane analysis (Hillier and McDonnell 2011).

Pharmacological and metabolic studies in animals suggest that alcohol, phenobarbital, chlorpromazine, diazepam, and ACTH antagonists retard central compensation, whereas caffeine, betahistine, acetyl-DL-leucine, amphetamines, and glucocorticoids accelerate it (overview in Dutia 2010). It has not yet been sufficiently investigated whether these drugs influence the central compensation in humans and if so, how much.

2.3.4   Pragmatic Therapy

As explained above, the treatment of acute vestibular neuritis is based on three therapeutic principles: (1) symptomatic therapy, (2) causal therapy, and (3) improvement of central vestibular compensation.

2.3.4.1 Symptomatic Therapy

In the acute phase during the first 1–3 days, 100 mg dimenhydrinate (one to three suppositories per day) or other antivertiginous drugs (Table 1.11, p.48) can be given to suppress nausea and vomiting. Drugs should be stopped as soon as the patient no longer vomits, as they prolong the time required to achieve central compensation (see above).

2.3.4.2 Causal Therapy

Brief treatment with corticosteroids (methylprednisolone, initially 100 mg/day; dose is tapered off by 20 mg every 4th day) significantly improves peripheral vestibular function (Strupp et al. 2004). With this therapy, the proportion of patients with a functional improvement of the affected labyrinth is significantly increased from 39 to 62 %.

2.3.4.3 Improvement of Central Vestibular Compensation

A gradual program of physical exercise under the supervision of a physiotherapist improves the central vestibular compensation of a peripheral deficit. First, static stabilization is concentrated on, and then dynamic exercises are done for head-movements, balance control and gaze stabilization during eye–head–body movements. It is important that exercises for equilibrium and balance successively increase in degree of difficulty above normal levels, both with and without visual stabilization. The efficacy of physiotherapy in improving central vestibulospinal compensation in patients with vestibular neuritis has been proven in a prospective, randomized controlled clinical study (Strupp et al. 1998) and a Cochrane analysis (Hillier and McDonnell 2011).

Ineffective Therapy

Treatment with measures to improve circulation (vasodilators, low-molecular-weight dextrans, hydroxyethyl starches, local anesthetics, or inhibitors of the ganglion stellatum) is ineffective.

2.3.5 Differential Diagnosis and Clinical Problems

The diagnosis of vestibular neuritis is a diagnosis of exclusion. Other peripheral vestibular as well as central vestibular disorders must be considered: attacks of Menière's disease that last a maximum of 1 day, vestibular migraine, vestibular paroxysmia, and vestibular pseudoneuritis due to a brainstem or cerebellar lesion.

Any of the specific accompanying symptoms (see below), the duration and the recurrence of complaints, as well as the careful clinical examination and in unclear cases additional laboratory tests (CCT, MRI, Doppler, CSF tap, evoked potentials) also prove useful:

- An initially burning pain and blisters, as well as hearing disorders and facial paresis, are typical of herpes zoster oticus (Ramsay–Hunt syndrome).
- Cogan's syndrome (mostly in young women, relatively rare) is an autoimmune disease characterized by three signs: interstitial keratitis ("red eye"), audiological symptoms, and vestibular symptoms or deficits which often show rapid progress.
- Brainstem signs usually occur with lacunar infarctions or multiple sclerosis plaques in the entry zone of the eighth cranial nerve or vestibulocerebellum ("vestibular pseudoneuritis"). The latter is clinically characterized by incomplete caloric hyporesponsiveness and in addition central ocular motor signs (see below).

Peripheral vestibular neuritis can be differentiated from central vestibular pseudoneuritis with a sensitivity and specificity of 92 %, even without MR imaging by using multivariable regression based on five clinical signs (Cnyrim et al. 2008):

- Skew deviation (vertical divergence, i.e., one eye above the other as a component of the ocular tilt reaction)
- Normal head-impulse test
- Central fixation nystagmus
- Gaze-evoked nystagmus in the opposite direction to that of spontaneous nystagmus
- Saccadic smooth pursuit

Concretely, this means that a patient with the above mentioned "central signs," a nonpathological head-impulse test, and a nystagmus that cannot be suppressed by visual fixation has a central disorder in the sense of a vestibular pseudoneuritis. The significance of the head-impulse test for the differential diagnosis has also been stressed in other studies (Newman-Toker et al. 2008; Kim and Lee 2012): acute vestibular vertigo with spontaneous nystagmus and a normal head-impulse test indicates a central origin. The findings are supported by a prospective study in 100 patients with acute vertigo in more than 95 % of the cases (Kattah et al. 2009).

In 10–15 % of patients with vestibular neuritis, a typical BPPV develops in the affected ear within a few weeks. It is possible that the otoconia become loose during the additional inflammation, and this eventually results in canalolithiasis. Patients should be warned about this possible complication because there are therapeutic liberatory maneuvers that can quickly free the patient of these complaints (see Sect. 2.2). A second important complication is that vestibular neuritis can develop into a somatoform phobic postural vertigo (see Sect. 5.2). The traumatic experience of a persisting (organic) rotatory vertigo leads to fearful introspection that results in a somatoform, fluctuating postural vertigo, which is reinforced by specific situations and culminates in a phobic avoidance behavior.

2.4 Menière's Disease

2.4.1 Patient History

Menière's disease is characterized by recurrent attacks of vertigo lasting several minutes to hours with hearing loss, tinnitus, and a feeling of fullness in the affected ear. Single attacks usually have no antecedent signs or recognizable precipitating factors. They occur both in daytime and at night. Approximately one-third of patients, however, report that an increase in tinnitus and in ear pressure and hearing loss precede the abrupt vertigo attack. Monosymptomatic attacks that are purely cochlear or vestibular can occur, particularly at the beginning of Menière's disease. During the course of the disease, most patients develop a progressive persistent hypoacusis of the affected ear.

2.4.2 Clinical Syndrome and Course

Menière's disease is typically a combination of abruptly occurring attacks with vestibular and/or cochlear symptoms with fluctuating, slowly progressive hearing loss; tinnitus; and in the course of time vestibular deficits.

The American Academy of Ophthalmology and Otolaryngology, Head and Neck Surgery formulated the following diagnostic criteria in 1995:

Certain Menière's disease

- Histopathological confirmation of endolymphatic hydrops
- Symptoms as in "definite Menière's disease" criteria

Definite Menière's disease

- Two or more attacks of vertigo, each lasting more than 20 min
- Audiometrically documented hearing loss in at least one examination
- Tinnitus or aural fullness in the affected ear
- Other causes excluded

Probable Menière's disease

- One vertigo episode
- Audiometrically documented hearing loss in at least one examination
- Tinnitus or aural fullness in the affected ear
- Other causes excluded

Possible Menière's disease

- Attacks of vertigo but without documented hearing loss
- Sensorineural hearing loss, fluctuating or fixed, with postural vertigo, but without definite episodes of vertigo
- Other causes excluded.

These recommendations definitely require improvement (Stapleton and Mills 2008) in at least two respects: as regards the clinical confirmation of the diagnosis and its distinction from other differential diagnoses, since there are several overlaps, e.g., with vestibular migraine, perilymph fistula, vestibular paroxysmia, and episodic ataxia type 2 (see Sect. 2.4.5). The diagnosis is frequently difficult or remains uncertain, especially in cases of a monosymptomatic beginning with isolated sudden deafness or isolated attacks of vertigo.

During the attack, there is first a unilateral short vestibular excitation, then a longer-lasting vestibulocochlear deficit with the following clinical findings:

- During the initial vestibular excitation: rotatory vertigo and nystagmus to the side of the affected labyrinth (i.e., an excitation-induced nystagmus) and a tendency to fall to the side of the unaffected ear.
- During the vestibular deficit: rotatory vertigo and nystagmus to the side of the healthy labyrinth (a deficit-induced nystagmus) and deviation of gait and a tendency to fall to the side of the affected ear.
- In addition, there are cochlear symptoms in the form of tinnitus, reduced hearing as well as pressure, and a feeling of fullness in the affected ear.

According to the diagnostic criteria above, an audiological examination is necessary, and complementary vestibular diagnostic measures are helpful. Audiometry usually detects a deafness of the inner ear for low tones (Savastano et al. 2006). In most, but not all, cases, audiological testing also helps differentiate between Menière's disease and vestibular migraine (Battista 2004; Cha et al. 2007; De Valck et al. 2007). The acoustic evoked potentials (AEP) indicate inner-ear deafness. By means of video-oculography with caloric testing, it is possible to document the peripheral vestibular deficit and its course. These procedures as well as vestibular-evoked myogenic potentials (VEMP) allow us to identify the affected ear and determine if a bilateral Menière's disease is present.

The lifetime prevalence of Menière's disease is around 0.5 % (Neuhauser 2007); this means that about one million Europeans are affected. Menière's disease is the second most frequent cause of peripheral vestibular vertigo after BPPV. The onset of the disease is usually between the fourth and sixth decades (men are affected somewhat more often than women); it rarely occurs in childhood (Choung et al. 2006).

The disease begins in one ear with very irregular attacks that at first increase then decrease again in frequency. The other ear can also become affected over time. The longer one follows these patients, the more often one sees a bilateral involvement (Nabi and Parnes 2009). In the early stage of the disease (up to 2 years), 15 % of the cases are bilateral. After 10 years, about 35 % develop a bilateral form and after 20 years, up to 47 %

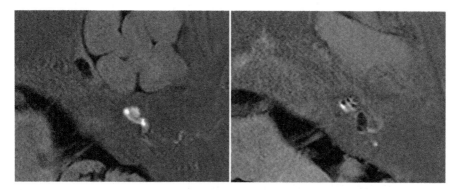

Fig. 2.10 Image of endolymph hydrops by means of high-resolution MRI of the petrous bone 24 h after transtympanic injection of gadolinium in a healthy subject (*left*) and a patient with Menière's disease (*right*). The black areas are due to the enlargement of the endolymphatic space, i.e., endolymphatic hydrops (Images supplied courtesy of Robert Gürkov et al. (2012))

(Huppert et al. 2010). This also explains why the disease is the second most frequent cause of a bilateral vestibulopathy (Zingler et al. 2007a). At first, the patients are without symptoms in the interval between attacks, and then they develop increasing buzzing sounds in the ear, reduced hearing (loss not only of deep tones) and postural imbalance. Compared with other inner-ear diseases, these symptoms are unusually variable in their extent. In the meantime, it is well known that the course of the disease in many patients is benign (Huppert et al. 2010): the frequency of attacks declines in the first 5–10 years.

2.4.3 Etiology, Pathophysiology, and Therapeutic Principles

Despite many studies, the etiology and pathophysiology of Menière's disease have not yet been fully clarified (overview in Minor et al. 2004; Semaan et al. 2005; Sajjadi and Paparella 2008). The pathognomonic histopathological finding is an endolymphatic hydrops (Merchant et al. 2005). This can nowadays be visualized by high-resolution MRI after transtympanic injection of gadolinium (see Fig. 2.10) (Gürkov et al. 2012). Pathophysiologically the hydrops develops as a result of a relatively too high production and/or a too low resorption of endolymph. The elevated endolymphatic pressure causes the membrane separating the endolymph space from the perilymph space to rupture or the voltage-sensitive unselective cation channels to open (Yeh et al. 1998). This results in an elevation of the potassium concentration in the perilymph space and thus potassium-induced depolarization, which first leads to excitation and then depolarization. The causes of endolymphatic hydrops are many; they range from autoimmunological and infectious diseases (Selmani et al. 2005) to hypotheses that ion-channel-related diseases (Gates 2005) or aquaporins (Ishiyama et al. 2006) can play an important role. Furthermore, on the basis of familial clusters (Frykholm et al. 2006; Klockars and Kentala 2007), genetic factors are now being discussed which are supported by linkage analyses (Klar et al. 2006).

The primary goal of therapy for Menière's disease is to prevent attacks in order to also prevent the progression of vestibulocochlear deficits. More than 2,000 papers have been published on the treatment of the disease so far. Accordingly the spectrum of therapy recommendations ranges from a salt-free diet, diuretics, transtympanic administration of gentamicin, steroids, or betahistine to different operative procedures (overview in Minor et al. 2004). The transtympanic instillation of gentamicin and steroids as well as high-dose, long-term administration of betahistine dihydrochloride (at least 3×48 mg/day for 12 months) has been reported to have positive effects on the frequency of attacks (overview in Strupp et al. 2007; Strupp and Brandt 2013).

2.4.3.1 Transtympanic instillation of gentamicin

The effect of gentamicin is based on the direct damage it causes to vestibular type 1 hair cells (Carey et al. 2002; Ishiyama et al. 2007; Selimoglu 2007). When this treatment was first introduced, the patients received gentamicin until vestibular function failed. In this way, freedom from attacks was achieved in most cases but at the cost of a clear inner-ear hypoacusis in more than 50 % of these cases. When it was proven that the ototoxic effect of the aminoglycosides began only after a definite delay the therapy regimen was changed to either single injections, each at least 4 weeks apart, or a single injection and subsequently regular follow-ups. Only if further attacks occurred were more injections given (Lange et al. 2004; De Stefano et al. 2007).

Two prospective double-blind randomized controlled studies have shown efficacy for vertigo (Postema et al. 2008; Stokroos and Kingma 2004). These results have been supported by a Cochrane analysis (Pullens and van Benthem 2011).

The fundamental problem of treatment with aminoglycosides is hearing damage, which affects at least 20 % of the patients (Colletti et al. 2007; Flanagan et al. 2006). For this reason, only patients with obvious preexisting hearing damage should actually receive this treatment. To make matters worse, many patients develop a bilateral Menière's disease after a period of 10 years (Takumida et al. 2006; Huppert et al. 2010).

2.4.3.2 Transtympanic Administration of Glucocorticoids

The effects of transtympanic injections of dexamethasone were examined in a retrospective study involving 34 patients (Barrs 2004). After 1 week of administering injections (10 mg/ml per injection), only 24 % of the patients showed a relevant improvement; another 24 % improved over the course of time, so that half of those treated profited. The treatment was well tolerated. A controlled, prospective, double-blind study showed an improvement of the attacks of vertigo in 82 % as opposed to 57 % in the placebo group (Garduno-Anaya et al. 2005). According to a Cochrane analysis (Phillips and Westerberg 2011), the study of Garduno-Anaya is so far the only study that has been performed with precise methods. Thus, the indications of the efficacy of transtympanal administration of glucocorticoids are limited. In a prospective, controlled randomized study, the effect of

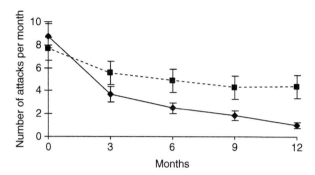

Fig. 2.11 Effect of betahistine dihydrochloride (low dosage (■), 16 or 24 mg 3× daily, compared to a higher dosage (♦), 48 mg 3× daily) on the frequency of attacks of Menière's disease in 112 patients during an open observation of therapy. The mean number of attacks per month (±SEM) is given during the 3 months before beginning therapy and during the therapy. After 12 months of treatment, the arithmetic mean or the median of the attacks declined in the group on the lower dosage from 7.6 (4.5) to 4.4 (2.0) ($p < 0.0001$); the number of attacks in the group on the higher dosage fell from 8.8 (5.5) to 1.0 (0.0) ($p < 0.0001$). The number of attacks after 12 months was significantly lower in the group on the higher dosage than in the group on the lower dosage (p12M = 0.0002) (reproduced with permission from Strupp et al. (2008))

intratympanic gentamicin was compared with that of dexamethasone: gentamicin was superior, reducing vertigo attacks by 93 % compared with 61 % with dexamethasone (Casani et al. 2012).

2.4.3.3 Betahistine

Meta-analyses show that betahistine evidently has a prophylactic effect on attacks of Menière's disease (Claes and Van-de-Heyning 1997; James and Thorp 2005; Strupp et al. 2007), although no state-of-the-art placebo-controlled, double-blind study has yet been published. Betahistine is a weak H1 agonist and H3 antagonist. It improves the microcirculation of the inner ear by acting on the precapillary sphincter of the stria vascularis (Dziadziola et al. 1999; Ihler et al. 2012). In this way, it can normalize the imbalance between production and resorption of endolymph. On the basis of clinical experience with a dosing regimen of 3 × 48 mg betahistine dihydrochloride per day, an open pilot study was performed in 112 patients. It showed that the higher doses were significantly superior to the usual dosage of 3 × 16–3 × 24 mg per day. After 12 months, the average number of attacks declined from 7.6/month to 4.4 in the low-dosage group and from 8.8 to 1.0 in the high-dosage group ($p = 0.0002$ in the group comparison) (Fig. 2.11) (Strupp et al. 2008). If the patients do not respond sufficiently after 3 months on a dosage of 3 × 48 mg per day, it can be successively increased in individual cases up to 480 mg per day (Lezius et al. 2011) or even 720 mg per day (Strupp et al. 2011). The goal of therapy is freedom from attacks for at least 6 months; then the dosage can be slowly reduced again to a maintenance dosage.

2.4.4 Pragmatic Therapy

2.4.4.1 Treatment of Attacks

The acute attack is limited. Vertigo and nausea can be reduced by antivertiginous drugs used in other acute disorders of labyrinthine function, e.g., 100 mg dimenhydrinate as suppository or infusion ($1-3 \times 100$ mg per day) or in severe cases benzodiazepine.

2.4.4.2 Prophylactic Therapy

The goal of prophylactic treatment is to reduce the endolymphatic hydrops in order to prevent attacks and the progression of vestibulocochlear deficits. If patients have one or more attacks per month, a prophylactic therapy is indicated.

- Betahistine dihydrochloride, 3×2 tablets of 24 mg each per day, i.e., 3×48 mg per day, for at least 12 months. If the patient is free of attacks for at least 6 months, the dose can be slowly tapered (depending on the course by 1 tablet every 3 months). This is a long-term treatment. The recommendations are based on the above-mentioned open pilot study (Strupp et al. 2008). If the frequency of attacks does not decline after 3 months, the dosage can be successively increased (up to 30 tablets per day, each 24 mg). If the patient is free of attacks for at least 6 months, the daily dosage can reasonably be again successively tapered by 24 mg every 3 months.

The following rare therapy is indicated for drug-resistant cases of Menière's disease with frequent attacks and inner-ear hypoacusis in which the affected side has been identified:

- Transtympanic instillation of ototoxic antibiotics (1–2 ml of gentamicin in a concentration of 20–40 mg/ml) at intervals of at least 4 weeks. The dosing interval should depend on the efficacy. According to meta-analyses, the success rate of the treatment lies between 39 and 95 % (Cohen-Kerem et al. 2004; Strupp et al. 2007). Earlier the instillations were given daily until it was proven that the ototoxic effects of gentamicin can appear with a delay (Magnusson and Padoan 1991). This is why nowadays single instillations are recommended but generally only at intervals of at least 4 weeks (Postema et al. 2008; Pullens and van Benthem 2011; Stokroos and Kingma 2004).

2.4.4.3 Treatment of Tumarkin's Otolithic Crises (Vestibular Drop Attacks)

Tumarkin's otolithic crises, i.e., vestibular drop attacks, are characterized by sudden, recurring falls without loss of consciousness, probably due to fluctuations of endolymphatic pressure in connection with unilateral otolith dysfunction and loss of vestibulospinal tonus. About 3–7 % of patients with Menière's disease report having drop attacks in both the early and late course of the disease (Baloh et al. 1990). Drop attacks are an extreme impairment of patients' everyday life. Moreover, they are dangerous because of the high rate of injuries. Depending on clinical judgement as to the severity of the disorder—in case the high-dosage treatment with betahistine did not result in improvement—intratympanic gentamicin treatment can be administered with success. The prerequisite for such treatment is that the causative ear can be definitely identified (e.g., by audiogram, caloric testing, or VEMP).

Ineffective Treatment of Menière's Disease

Meta-analyses have shown that a salt-free diet (Strupp et al. 2007) or diuretics (Thirlwall and Kundu 2006) have no significant effect. Saccotomy is also ineffective, as was pointed out in a Cochrane analysis (Pullens et al. 2013). Thus, these procedures are nowadays obsolete just like selective neurectomy, which was widely used in the past.

2.4.5   Differential Diagnosis and Clinical Problems

The typical patient history is the key to the diagnosis. The otoneurological and neuro-ophthalmological examination during the attack-free interval reveals fluctuating, overall progressive hearing loss and a peripheral vestibular deficit (depending on whether it is unilateral or bilateral). An early diagnosis is often difficult, since the onset of Menière's disease shows the classic triad in only 20 % of patients; in 40 %, a sudden unilateral deafness at the onset; and in the remaining 40 %, a rotatory vertigo lasting minutes to several hours.

The two most important diseases for the differential diagnosis during the first attacks of Menière's disease are vestibular neuritis (Sect. 2.3) and in case of recurrent attacks, vestibular migraine (Sect. 3.2). The duration of the attacks is helpful for differentiating Menière's disease from vestibular neuritis: whereas in Menière's disease they generally last several hours and at most one day, in vestibular neuritis, they last several days. The accompanying symptoms are also helpful for the differential diagnosis:

- "Ear symptoms" in Menière's disease
- Inflamed eye signs, hearing disturbances and vestibular dysfunction in Cogan's syndrome
- Hearing disorders and possibly central signs in infarctions of the AICA/labyrinthine artery.

Central disorders of vestibular function also occur after lacunar infarctions or MS plaques in the area of the entry zone of the eighth cranial nerve ("fascicular lesion") or vestibulo-cerebellum (vestibular pseudoneuritis), or in vestibular migraine. Since a caloric hyporeactivity occurs in the majority of the above-named diseases (Sect. 2.3), this cannot be used in the differential diagnosis.

In cases of recurring attacks, vestibular migraine is the important differential diagnosis. These attacks can be short or also last for several hours (Sect. 3.2). Here it is important to stress that 60 % of patients with Menière's disease also fulfill the diagnostic criteria for vestibular migraine; this is conversely true of patients with vestibular migraine (Radtke et al. 2002). A pathogenetic association of the two diseases is likely.

Signs that the attack is a vestibular migraine are (1) central ocular motor disorders during the attack or the attack-free interval (also typical for episodic ataxia type 2, Sect. 3.2.5 and 6.1.4), (2) the absence of progressive hearing loss despite many attacks, (3) the association with other neurological symptoms such as numbness of the face or speech disorders (basilar type migraine), (4) head and neck pain, and (5) response to prophylactic treatment for migraine.

Signs indicating Menière's disease are audiological deficits and also the typical feeling of pressure on the affected ear.

Frequently, the diagnosis can only be made on the basis of the course of the illness and the response to therapy. A portion of the patients must be treated prophylactically for Menière's disease as well as vestibular migraine before they are free of symptoms.

Rare, sudden recurrent falls, so-called vestibular drop attacks (Tumarkin's otolithic crisis), which occur in the early or late stages of Menière's disease without definite triggers, antecedent signs, or disturbances of consciousness, are difficult to differentiate from drop attacks caused by vertebrobasilar ischemia (Baloh et al. 1990).

Vestibular paroxysmia, which is caused by neurovascular compression (Sect. 2.5), is also characterized by recurrent attacks with vertigo and/or occasionally other ear symptoms. These attacks typically last only seconds in contrast to Menière's disease.

2.5   Vestibular Paroxysmia

2.5.1   Patient History

The main symptoms of vestibular paroxysmia are brief attacks of rotatory or postural vertigo lasting seconds to a few minutes, with or without ear symptoms (tinnitus and hypoacusis). In some patients, the attacks frequently depend on certain positions of the head; they can occasionally be induced by hyperventilation. Hearing loss and tinnitus can also be present during the attack-free intervals.

2.5.2   Clinical Aspects and Course

Vestibular paroxysmia is suspected if brief and frequent attacks of vertigo are accompanied by the following features (Brandt and Dieterich 1994; Hüfner et al. 2008a):

- Short attacks of rotatory or postural vertigo last for seconds to minutes with instability of posture and gait.
- Attacks may be triggered by particular head positions and hyperventilation, or be influenced by changing the head position.

- Unilateral hypoacusis or tinnitus occurs during the attacks, occasionally or permanently.
- In the course of the disease, measurable vestibular and/or cochlear deficits increase during the attack and are less pronounced during the attack-free interval (neurophysiological function tests used include audiogram, acoustic-evoked potentials, caloric testing, test for subjective visual vertical).
- Attacks are improved or lessened by administering carbamazepine (even low dosage effective).
- No central vestibular/ocular motor disorders or brainstem signs are present.

Approximately 20 % of patients undergoing ocular motor and functional testing of the eighth cranial nerve exhibit signs of a unilateral vestibular hypofunction (head-shaking nystagmus, pathological head-impulse test). In some of the patients, spontaneous nystagmus can be provoked by hyperventilation (Hüfner et al. 2008a).

Conclusions can be drawn from the type of complaints—vestibular (originating from the canals or otolith organs) or cochlear symptoms—about the portion of the nerve affected. If there is a combination of symptoms of various nerves, the site of the lesion can possibly be deduced. Thus, for example, simultaneously occurring symptoms of the seventh and eighth cranial nerves (with contraction of the frontal muscle, vertigo, and slightly staggered double images; Straube et al. 1994) indicate an irritation of both nerves in the internal acoustic meatus, where both lie in close proximity to each other. Finally, an analogous clinical syndrome with relapsing tinnitus has been described (Russell and Baloh 2009). It can be equally a sign of an excitation as well as of an inhibition.

In a study on 32 patients with vestibular paroxysmia, neurovascular compression in the terminal area of the vestibulocochlear nerve was detected in 95 % of the affected patients. For this reason, a high-resolution MRI with CISS sequences of the brainstem can support the diagnosis. A bilateral neurovascular compression was found in 42 % of the patients (Hüfner et al. 2008a). Since such neurovascular compressions are known to also occur in healthy subjects, they can be diagnosed as pathological only in connection with the corresponding accompanying clinical symptoms (see Table 2.3). In trigeminal neuralgia, high-resolution diffusion tensor imaging revealed significant lower anisotropy and a higher apparent diffusion coefficient in the affected trigeminal root, which correlates with structural atrophic nerve changes (Leal et al. 2011). Comparable findings are not yet available for the eighth nerve due to methodological limitations by the short course of the eighth nerve from the brainstem to the internal acoustic meatus and the adjacent temporal bone. A cranial MRI should also be performed to exclude the presence of a tumor in the area of the cerebellar pontine angle, arachnoid cysts, megalodolichobasilaris, brainstem plaques in MS (paroxysmal brainstem attacks), or other brainstem lesions.

There seem to be two peaks of frequency: one that begins early in cases of vertebrobasilar vascular anomalies and a second between the ages of 40 and 70 in cases of vascular elongation due to increasing atherosclerosis and stronger pulsations due to hypertension of old age. The course is generally chronic. Men are affected twice as often as women.

Table 2.3 Diagnostic criteria for vestibular paroxysmia

Definite vestibular paroxysmia

At least five attacks and the patient also fulfills criteria A–E

A. Vertigo spells lasting seconds to minutes. The individual attack is self-limiting and subsides without specific therapeutic intervention

B. One or several of the following provoking factors induce the attacks:
   1. Occurring in rest
   2. Certain head/body positions
   3. Changes in head/body positions (not BPPV-specific positioning maneuvers)

C. None or one or several of the following characteristics during the attacks:
   1. Disturbance of stance
   2. Disturbance of gait
   3. Unilateral tinnitus
   4. Unilateral pressure/numbness in or around the ear
   5. Unilaterally reduced hearing

D. One or several of the following additional diagnostic criteria:
   1. Neurovascular cross-compression demonstrated on MRI (CISS or FIESTA sequence, TOF MR angiography)
   2. Hyperventilation-induced nystagmus as measured by video-oculography
   3. Increase of vestibular deficit at follow-up investigations
   4. Treatment response to antiepileptics (not applicable at first consultation)

E. The symptoms cannot be explained by another disease.

Probable vestibular paroxysmia

At least five attacks and the patient fulfills criterion A and at least three of criteria B–E

From Hüfner et al. (2008a); modified after a table in Brandt and Dieterich (1994)
BPPV benign paroxysmal positioning vertigo, *CISS* constructive interference in steady-state sequence, *FIESTA* fast imaging employing steady-state acquisition sequence, *TOF* time of flight

2.5.3 Etiology, Pathophysiology, and Therapeutic Principles

As in trigeminal neuralgia, hemifacial spasm, glossopharyngeal neuralgia, or myokymia of the superior oblique muscle (Hüfner et al. 2008b), it is assumed that a neurovascular cross-compression of the eighth cranial nerve is the cause of these short, second-long episodes of vertigo (Møller et al. 1986; Brandt and Dieterich 1994; Strupp et al. 2013). Aberrant, in part arteriosclerotically elongated and dilated, and consequently more pulsating arteries in the cerebellopontine angle are thought to be the pathophysiological cause of a segmental pressure-induced lesion with demyelination of the central (oligodendroglia) myelin. A loop of the AICA seems to be involved most often (Fig. 2.12), less often the PICA, the vertebral artery or a vein. The symptoms are triggered by direct pulsatile compression and/or ephaptic discharges, i.e., pathological paroxysmal interaxonal transmission between neighboring and in part demyelinated axons. Another cause under discussion is central hyperactivity in the nucleus, which is induced and maintained by the compression. Finally, in addition to elongation and increased looping, a vascular malformation or arterial ectasia of the posterior fossa can also cause the nerve compression.

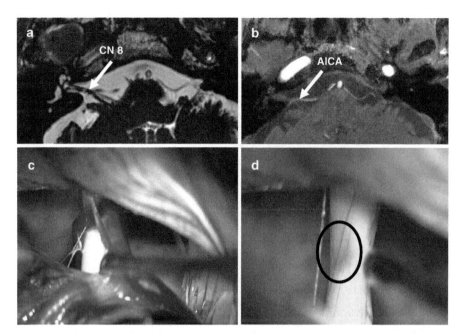

Fig. 2.12 Cranial MRI (**a**, constructive interference in steady-state sequence; **b**, time-of-flight sequence) shows contact between the right eighth cranial nerve (*CN 8*, *arrow* in **a**) and the anterior inferior cerebellar artery (*AICA*, *arrow* in **b**). Intraoperative micrographs demonstrate the vascular contact (**c**) and the considerable compression of the eighth nerve after removal of the arteries (**d**, *circle*) (Reproduced with permission from Strupp et al. (2013))

This etiology was previously connected with the so-called disabling positional vertigo (Jannetta et al. 1984), a very heterogeneous syndrome of vertigo with symptoms of various durations (from seconds to days), various characteristic features (rotatory or postural vertigo, light-headedness or gait instability without vertigo), and varying accompanying symptoms. As these vague descriptions also applied to patients with BPPV (Sect. 2.2), Menière's disease (Sect. 2.4), bilateral vestibulopathy (Sect. 2.6), or somatoform phobic postural vertigo (Sect. 5.1), the clinical definition was subsequently made more precise (Brandt and Dieterich 1994).

Despite signs of an arterial (rarely venous) compression of the eighth cranial nerve, which are visible in MRI (with CISS or FIESTA and TOF MR angiography; Fig. 2.12), larger prospective clinical studies are still lacking as to how frequently such neurovascular contacts can also be imaged in healthy subjects. It is unclear which region of the myelin sheath of the vestibulocochlear nerve is the most vulnerable (distance measured precisely in millimeters from the nerve exit zone out of the brainstem) (Fig. 2.13). However, it can be assumed that it is the long intracisternal course, which is surrounded by central myelin of the oligodendrocytes. This corresponds to the first 15 mm after the nerve exits (Lang 1982).

Occasionally, vertigo attacks lasting seconds and caused by head movements point to an arachnoid cyst that stretches the vestibulocochlear nerve (Arbusow et al.

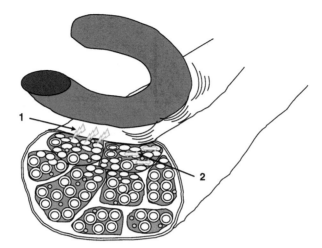

Fig. 2.13 Pathophysiology of vestibular paroxysmia on analogy to other neurovascular compression syndromes. *1* shows the schematic drawing of the ephaptic activation of axons in the demyelinated neurons caused by pulsatile compression, and *2* indicates schematically a place of intraaxonal ephaptic discharge, i.e., pathologically paroxysmal interaxonal transmission between neighboring and in part demyelinated axons (Reproduced with permission from Hüfner et al. (2009))

1998a). This pathogenesis can result in a combination of longer-lasting conduction-block symptoms in one direction (hours to days) with additional symptoms of head movement-induced excitations (for seconds) in the opposite direction.

2.5.4 Pragmatic Therapy

2.5.4.1 Medical Treatment

A therapeutic approach with a low dosage of carbamazepine (200–600 mg/day) or oxcarbazepine (300–600 mg/day) is expedient, and moreover, a positive response is diagnostic. A study on the course of the disease in 32 patients over a 3-year period revealed a significant and continuing decrease in the attack frequency up to 10 % of the initial value as well as a reduction in the intensity and duration of the attacks (Hüfner et al. 2008a). In case of intolerance, phenytoin, gabapentin, and valproic acid are possible alternatives; however, there are no study data yet available.

2.5.4.2 Surgical Treatment

Despite the report of partial successes (Møller et al. 1986) and clinically well-documented single cases (Strupp et al. 2013), operative microvascular decompression should be avoided because, on the one hand, there is the risk of a brainstem infarction due to intra- or postoperative vasospasm (ca. 3–5 %), and, on the other, it is frequently difficult to determine the affected side with enough certainty. However, if there are additional causes, such as the abovementioned arachnoid cyst in the cerebellar pontine angle, the operation is recommended, as drug therapy only rarely leads to the absence of symptoms.

Ineffective Treatment

Treatments with circulation-promoting measures and antivertiginous drugs are ineffective.

2.5.5 Differential Diagnosis and Clinical Problems

Important differential diagnoses are:

- BPPV
- Paroxysmal brainstem attacks
- Vestibular migraine
- Phobic postural vertigo
- Panic attacks
- Vertebral artery occlusion syndrome (dependent on head position)
- Central positional/positioning nystagmus.

The differential diagnosis is generally straightforward, because of the characteristic brevity (seconds up to a few minutes, very seldom many hours) and the frequently recurring attacks of vertigo. Only paroxysmal brainstem attacks with vertigo, dysarthria, and, for example, ataxia can be difficult to distinguish, as they too respond to low dosages of carbamazepine. It has been shown that they are caused by a midbrain lesion due to MS plaques or lacunar infarctions (Li et al. 2011), which also leads to ephaptic discharges of neighboring fibers of the brainstem paths. In such cases, the use of MRI with thin brainstem slices is expedient for establishing the diagnosis.

BPPV due to canalolithiasis can be diagnosed by the typical crescendo–decrescendo nystagmus (Sect. 2.2) caused by the positioning maneuver. These typical characteristics do not occur with vestibular paroxysmia and are not triggered as regularly by positioning.

2.6 Bilateral Vestibulopathy

2.6.1 Patient History

Key symptoms of bilateral vestibulopathy are:

- Movement-dependent dizziness, postural imbalance and unsteadiness of gait and stance (exacerbated in the dark and on unlevel ground) but free of symptoms when sitting or lying

- Blurred vision when walking and during head movements (oscillopsia) (in about 40 % of patients)
- Spatial memory and navigation impairment

Patients mostly complain about postural imbalance, dizziness and gait unsteadiness when moving. They are typically free of symptoms under static conditions, i.e., when sitting or lying. About 40 % of those affected notice illusory movements of the surroundings (oscillopsia) while walking or running, and consequently, they can no longer read street signs or definitely identify the faces of people approaching them. Especially patients with sequential or "idiopathic" bilateral vestibulopathy may report attacks of spontaneous rotatory or postural vertigo in the initial phases, which can persist for several minutes or days. Evidently during these phases, the function of the vestibular system worsens on one side.

2.6.2   Clinical Aspects and Natural Course

Bilateral vestibular failure is the most frequent cause of movement-dependent postural vertigo in elderly patients (for relative frequency, see Table 1.1). However, it is often not diagnosed at all or diagnosed late. Clinical suspicion of a bilateral vestibulopathy is based on the above-mentioned key symptoms. The diagnosis is confirmed by testing the VOR and otolith function by a combination of:

- The head-impulse test (Halmagyi and Curthoys 1988) (see Fig. 1.14)
- The caloric test (see Fig. 1.20)
- Cervical and ocular vestibular-evoked myogenic potentials (see Fig. 1.26)

The head-impulse test reveals refixation saccades when the head is turned horizontally to the right and to the left; they indicate a high-frequency deficit of the VOR. If the result cannot be clinically evaluated with certainty, an examination with video-oculography should be performed to quantify the VOR amplification factor (the so-called VOR gain) (MacDougall et al. 2009). Caloric testing with recording of eye movements can be used for documentation purposes, measurements, or examination—above all in cases of differences between the two sides—and for testing the VOR in the low-frequency range. Testing of the VOR reveals three groups of patients: those with a combined high- and low-frequency deficit (the majority), those with only a high-frequency deficit, or those with only a low-frequency deficit (Kim et al. 2011b; Zingler et al. 2007a). Finally, dynamic visual acuity testing can be used to determine the reduction of the vision during head turns; it helps to establish a diagnosis (Vital et al. 2010). Otherwise, the ocular motor system is normal. Exceptions are patients with a combination of cerebellar ocular motor disorders (the so-called CANVAS) (see below). Tests of gait and stance with the eyes open are basically normal; only when the eyes are closed is there increased body instability during the Romberg test; this becomes more obvious during tandem standing, one-leg standing, as well as walking toe to heel. In the latter three tests, there is a danger of falling. Asymmetries of the vestibular function are observed when the patient walks straight ahead with closed eyes: the direction of gait deviation as a rule indicates the side most affected.

In the course of bilateral vestibulopathy, both labyrinths and vestibular nerves can be affected at the same time or sequentially; the disorder can be acute or slowly progressive, complete or incomplete, and with or without a difference in the side affected. Bilateral vestibulopathy can occur with or without associated hearing loss. As a rule, the diagnosis of bilateral vestibulopathy is made by testing the function of the horizontal canal pathways. An examination of cervical vestibular-evoked myogenic potentials revealed that the saccular function is less impaired than the canals (Zingler et al. 2008). However, there is evidently also a rare subcategory of bilateral sacculopathy in which the canal function is normal (Fujimoto et al. 2009).

A 5-year follow-up of more than 80 patients with bilateral vestibulopathy found that more than 80 % of the patients had no significant improvement of vestibular deficits regardless of etiology, type of course, sex, or age at first manifestation (Zingler et al. 2007b).

2.6.3 Pathophysiology, Etiology, and Therapeutic Principles

The key symptoms of bilateral vestibulopathy can be explained by the loss of vestibulo-ocular and vestibulospinal functions.

2.6.3.1 Unsteadiness of Posture and Gait as well as Postural Vertigo

Increased in the dark and on unlevel ground: Due to the redundant sensorimotor control of posture, the visual system can basically substitute for any defective regulation of postural control in light. The somatosensory system also contributes to the maintenance of balance, above all via the muscle spindle afferents and the mechanoreceptors of the skin. If the contribution of the visual system (in darkness or due to visual disorders) is reduced, gait imbalance increases until the patient experiences a tendency to fall. This is further intensified if the patient walks in the dark over unlevel or springy ground. A sensory polyneuropathy also reduces the somatosensory contribution to posture control and thereby exacerbates the symptoms of bilateral vestibulopathy.

2.6.3.2 Oscillopsia and Blurred Vision

During rapid head movements, the impaired VOR cannot maintain the target of gaze on the fovea, and thus, there is an involuntary movement of the image on the retina, which is experienced as an illusory movement that reduces the visual acuity. This symptom occurs in 40 % of the patients (Zingler et al. 2007a). Conversely, when head movements are slow, the smooth pursuit system is able to sufficiently stabilize the gaze in space, and no illusory movement or blurriness occurs.

2.6.3.3 Deficits of Spatial Memory and Navigation

An intact vestibular function is important for spatial orientation, spatial memory, and navigation (Smith 1997). Significant deficits of spatial memory and navigation as well as atrophy of the hippocampus were demonstrated in patients with bilateral vestibulopathy (Brandt et al. 2005). The other memory functions are not affected. In patients with unilateral labyrinthine failure, however, no disorders of spatial memory or atrophy of the hippocampus were found (Hüfner et al. 2007).

2.6.3.4 Etiology

The etiology of bilateral vestibulopathy remained unclear in 50 % of 255 patients (Zingler et al. 2007a). Most of them can be assumed to have a degenerative illness (see below). The three most frequent causes of bilateral vestibulopathy beyond that were (Zingler et al. 2007a):

- Ototoxic aminoglycosides (13 %)
- Menière's disease (7 %)
- Meningitis (5 %).

Other causes are bilateral vestibular schwannoma (neurofibromatosis type 2) or autoimmune diseases (Arbusow et al. 1998b) like Cogan's syndrome. In this syndrome, MRI shows typical hemorrhages and an enhanced uptake of contrast medium in the labyrinth and/or cochlea, indicating the activity of the disease. Patients with bilateral vestibulopathy frequently have a cerebellar syndrome and a downbeat nystagmus; the opposite is also true (Migliaccio et al. 2004; Zingler et al. 2007a; Wagner et al. 2008; Kirchner et al. 2011). Such cases probably involve a neurodegenerative illness that affects the vestibular ganglia cells and the cerebellum; it often occurs with an additional neuropathy: cerebellar ataxia with neuropathy and vestibular areflexia syndrome (CANVAS). This combination of symptoms occurs in up to 20 % of patients with bilateral vestibulopathy (Szmulewicz et al. 2011; Kirchner et al. 2011; Pothier et al. 2011).

2.6.3.5 Therapeutic Principles

Treatment of the various forms of bilateral vestibulopathy follows four lines of action:

1. Prophylaxis of progressive vestibular loss
2. Recovery of vestibular function
3. Promotion of central compensation (or substitution) of missing vestibular function with physical therapy
4. Informing and educating the patients

2.6.4 Pragmatic Therapy

2.6.4.1 Prevention

Prevention is most important for the group of patients with ototoxic labyrinthine damage, above all that due to aminoglycosides. Aminoglycoside therapy should be used only if strictly indicated and then only in a once-daily dose. Plasma levels should also be monitored. Patients with renal insufficiency, advanced age, or familial susceptibility to aminoglycoside ototoxicity are at particular risk. Ototoxic antibiotics should not be combined with other ototoxic substances, such as loop diuretics, as this can have a potentiating effect on inner-ear damage. Careful follow-ups of the hearing and vestibular function are necessary during treatment. However, the physician must remain vigilant, as the ototoxic effects of gentamicin have a delayed onset, often appearing only after days or weeks.

2.6.4.2 Recovery

Recovery of vestibular function is possible in post-meningitis cases due to a serous nonsuppurative labyrinthitis and in individual cases of autoimmunologically induced forms of inner-ear disease, which are diagnosed too infrequently. Although controlled prospective studies are lacking, immune treatment is theoretically expedient, if there are clinical signs of a systemic autoimmune disease or if antibodies against inner-ear structures are detected (Schüler et al. 2003; Deutschländer et al. 2005). Initially, corticosteroids can be tried (e.g., prednisolone in doses of 80 mg per day, tapered over ca. 3–4 weeks). In Cogan's syndrome, initially high doses of steroids (1 g i.v. daily for 5 days) can be given with subsequent dose reduction. If the response is inadequate or relapses occur, additional but temporary administration of azathioprine or cyclophosphamide is recommended. Besides this, treatment of the causative underlying disease (Table 2.2) is important and in individual cases also successful.

2.6.4.3 Physical Therapy of Stance and Gait

Patient response to physical therapy with gait and balance training is quite positive. This therapy alleviates the adaptation to loss of function by promoting visual and somatosensory substitution. Such substitution was proven with the help of functional imaging. It showed that larger portions of the visual and multisensory cortical areas of patients with bilateral vestibulopathy were activated during visual stimulation than in healthy persons of the same age (Dieterich et al. 2007). The efficacy of balance training was confirmed at least for patients with unilateral peripheral vestibular function disorders (Hillier and McDonnell 2011).

2.6.4.4   Informing and Educating the Patient

It is important to inform the patients carefully about the type, mechanism, and course of their illness. It is our experience that the diagnosis of a bilateral vestibulopathy is still established much too late, despite many visits to the physician, a fact that only intensifies the complaints of the patients. The disease has a pronounced negative impact on physical and social functioning, leading to deterioration of quality of life (Guinand et al. 2012). Frequently, these subjective complaints are reduced by simply informing the patient. In the long term, vestibular implants will be a therapeutic option. They have had promising results in animal studies (Merfeld and Lewis 2012) and in a pilot trial in humans (van de Berg et al. 2012).

2.6.5   Differential Diagnosis and Clinical Problems

Considerations for the differential diagnosis proceed along three lines:

- It is important to look for the causes listed in Table 2.4 if clinical signs of a bilateral vestibulopathy are present.
- It is necessary to differentiate the illness from other vestibular and non-vestibular diseases, which are also characterized by oscillopsia and/or instability of posture and gait (see Tables 1.6 and 1.7).

  - Cerebellar ataxias without bilateral vestibulopathy
  - Downbeat nystagmus syndrome
  - Phobic postural vertigo
  - Intoxications
  - Vestibular paroxysmia
  - Perilymph fistulas
  - Orthostatic hypotension
  - Orthostatic tremor
  - Ocular motor disorders (if oscillopsia is prominent)
  - Unilateral vestibular deficit

Table 2.4 Causes of bilateral vestibulopathy

Relatively frequent	Underlying cause
Idiopathic (>30 %)	
Ototoxicity	Gentamicin and other antibiotics
	Anticancer chemotherapy
	Loop diuretics
	Aspirin

Table 2.4 (continued)

Relatively frequent	Underlying cause
Cerebellar degeneration	Spinocerebellar degeneration/ataxia (SCA)
	CANVAS syndrome (cerebellar ataxia, neuropathy, vestibular areflexia syndrome)
	Multisystem atrophy
Meningitis or labyrinthitis	For example, Streptococci, Neisseria meningitis,
	Mycobacterium tuberculosis
	HIV-associated infections
Tumors	Neurofibromatosis type II (bilateral vestibular schwannomas)
	Non-Hodgkin's lymphoma
	Meningeosis carcinomatosa
	Infiltration of the skull base
Autoimmune disorders	Cogan's syndrome
	Neurosarcoidosis
	Behçet's disease
	Cerebral vasculitis
	Systemic lupus erythematosus
	Polychondritis
	Rheumatoid arthritis
	Polyarteritis nodosa
	Wegener's granulomatosis
	Giant cell arteritis
	Primary antiphospholipid syndrome
	Vitamin $B_{1, 6, 12}$ deficiency
	Hereditary sensory and autonomic neuropathy
Bilateral sequential vestibular neuritis	Herpes simplex virus type I
Bilateral Menière's disease	Endolymphatic hydrops
Relatively rare (or single cases)	
Congenital malformation	Usher's syndrome and other rare hereditary conditions
Other rare causes	Bilateral petrous bone fractures
	Paget's disease
	Macroglobulinemia
	Vertebrobasilar dolichoectasia
	Superficial siderosis

2.7 Perilymph Fistulas

2.7.1 Patient History

The cardinal symptoms of perilymph fistula (and superior canal dehiscence syndrome) are attacks of rotatory or postural vertigo caused by changes in pressure, for example, by coughing, pressing, sneezing, lifting, or loud noises and accompanied by illusory movements of the environment (oscillopsia) and instability of posture and gait with or without hearing disorders. The attacks, which can last seconds to days, can also occur during changes in the position of the head (e.g., when bending over) and when experiencing significant changes in altitude (e.g., mountain tours, flights). When taking the patient history, it is important to ask about traumas that could cause or trigger such attacks, for example, barotrauma, head trauma, ear trauma (also operations of the ear), or excessive Valsalva maneuvers due to lifting of heavy weights.

2.7.2 Clinical Aspects and Course

The clinical spectrum of complaints is characterized by a wide range of symptoms: episodic dizziness or rotatory vertigo of various intensity and duration (from seconds to days), oscillopsia, imbalance, and hearing loss. This variability depends on the site of the fistula, which can influence whether canal or otolith symptoms dominate. Consequently, it is difficult in many cases to establish the diagnosis. Rotatory vertigo suggests more the canal type, whereas postural to-and-fro vertigo suggests more the otolith type. Linear and rotatory nystagmus, oscillopsia, and a tendency to fall in a certain direction can occur in both forms. A fistula of the vertical canals is indicated by a vertical rotatory nystagmus, whereas a fistula of the horizontal canal is characterized by a linear horizontal nystagmus.

The following procedures are helpful for establishing the diagnosis:

- Provocation tests by changes in pressure
- Vestibular-evoked myogenic potentials
- High-resolution CT with imaging of the petrous bone
- Examination for a Tullio phenomenon.

The goal of provocation tests is to trigger attacks during observation (using Frenzel's glasses) or recording of the resulting eye movements with video-oculography, scanning laser ophthalmoscope, or the scleral-coil technique. Such provocative procedures include the Valsalva maneuver, the tragal pressure test, and examination with a Politzer balloon (see Fig. 1.4). The affected side can also be identified with the pressure test by means of the Politzer balloon or the tragal pressure test. A feeling of increased pressure in the ear, tinnitus, reduced hearing, or autophonia all can indicate the affected ear.

Imaging with computed tomography (CT) (in the form of high-resolution thin-slice CT; see Sect. 1.8) is an important tool, especially to prove the presence of the so-called superior semicircular canal dehiscence syndrome, the most frequent form of the perilymph fistulas (Fig. 2.14). ENT doctors use exploratory tympanoscopy when questions of hypermobility of the stapes, typically found with perilymph fistula of the anterior canal, or when fistulas of the round and oval windows are strongly suspected. This examination must be combined with the other above-mentioned procedures in order to make a correct diagnosis.

It has been proposed that the presence of perilymph proteins is a specific marker of perilymph fistula (Ikezono et al. 2010); however, the diagnostic selectivity of these proteins is ambiguous (Bachmann-Harilstad et al. 2011).

The Tullio phenomenon is characterized by the occurrence of vestibular otolith or canal symptoms caused by loud sounds. In this case, the attempt should be made

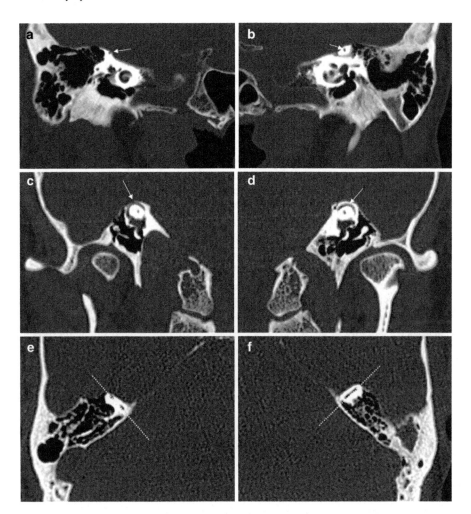

Fig. 2.14 High-resolution computed tomography scan of the petrous bone in a patient with a superior canal dehiscence syndrome (*left*) and a normal control (*right*); coronal slice (**a, b**), diagonal slice parallel to the axis of the anterior canal (**c, d**), and axial slice through the anterior canal (**e, f**). There is a bony defect in the apical part of in the right superior (anterior) canal extending toward the epidural space (**a, c,** *arrow*). For comparison, see healthy petrous bone (**b, d, f**) (courtesy of Dr. J. Linn)

to trigger vertigo and eye movements by exposing each of the patient's ears separately to loud sounds of different frequencies.

The incidence and prevalence of perilymph fistulas are not known because of the uncertain diagnosis; evidently they are relatively higher in childhood. However, perilymph fistulas can occur at any time in life, and there is no obvious preference for either sex. The course of the illness varies; sometimes the attacks are rare and sometimes frequent; as a rule, they can resolve spontaneously and there are symptom-free periods of various durations, which, however, can be reactivated by a new barotrauma.

2.7.2.1 Superior Canal Dehiscence Syndrome

In 1998, Minor and colleagues described a variant of a fistula caused by a dehiscence of the superior canal (Minor et al. 1998). In the meantime, this has become a well-established cause of episodic vertigo (Minor et al. 2005; Chien et al. 2011). This form is especially important, because it occurs frequently and is often overlooked. The main symptoms are rotatory or postural vertigo with oscillopsia induced by coughing or pressing and sometimes by loud sounds. In more than half of the patients, these complaints first occur after slight head concussion or barotrauma. Typically one can observe a Tullio phenomenon, a positive Hennebert sign (finger pressure on the external auditory canal causes eye movements), or a pathological Valsalva maneuver. Analysis of the eye movements in the attack reveals vertical-torsional nystagmus. The symptoms of the very rare dehiscence of the posterior canal (Chien et al. 2011) or the horizontal canal (Zhang et al. 2011) are similar.

The diagnosis of this internal perilymph fistula can be confirmed by thin-slice CT of the petrous bone (Fig. 2.14), which shows a bony apical defect of the superior, or rarely posterior or horizontal canal, and by 3-D analysis of eye movements induced by changes in pressure (Figs. 2.15 and 2.16). CT cannot confirm the diagnosis alone; a combination of tools and the presence of the clinical symptoms are necessary (Sequeira et al. 2011). The cervical vestibular-evoked myogenic potentials (cVEMP; see Fig. 1.26) electrophysiologically show a clearly reduced sensory threshold in the affected ear with 81 ± 9 dB compared to 99 ± 7 dB in the healthy ear (Watson et al. 2000; Minor 2005). Ocular vestibular-evoked myogenic potentials (Thabet et al. 2012; Niesten et al. 2013) and electrocochleographic examinations (Adams et al. 2011) can also support the diagnosis. About 8 % of the patients have primarily auditory symptoms; for example, they report that they can hear their pulse or their eye movements (Watson et al. 2000). This can be attributed to a higher sensitivity to the bone conduction of sound. The dehiscence syndrome also occurs in children, often at first only with auditory signs (Lee et al. 2011).

2.7.3 Pathophysiology and Therapeutic Principles

The perilymphatic and the endolymphatic space lie within the bony labyrinth. The border of tissue between the bony labyrinth and the middle ear forms the annular ligament of the base of the stapes and the membrane of the round window. These structures can rupture by stretching (blunt brain concussion), intracranial increase of pressure ("explosive pressure due to pressing," barotrauma), or a pressure-wave-induced trauma ("implosion"). Perilymph fistulas can develop in patients with congenitally weak membranes (thin bony apical cover of the superior canal) or a cholesteatoma after a bagatelle trauma, for example, sneezing or lifting heavy weights, and not be noticed.

At the root of all perilymph fistulas is pressure that is pathologically transmitted between the perilymphatic space and the middle ear or between the perilymphatic space and the intracranial space. They are caused by:

- A bony defect toward the epidural space in the "fistula" of the more frequent superior, less often of the horizontal and posterior canals. This bony defect leads

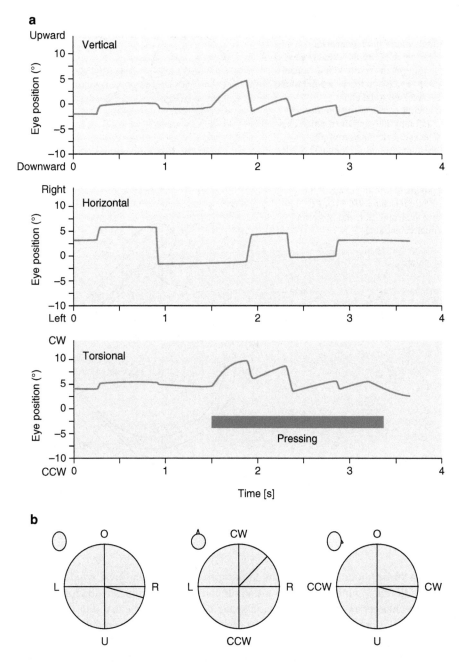

Fig. 2.15 (a) Original three-dimensional recording of vertical, horizontal, and torsional eye movements with the search-coil technique before, during, and after a Valsalva maneuver. Pressure-induced vertical (slow phase upward) and torsional (slow phase from viewpoint of the patient, counterclockwise) eye movements (*cw* clockwise, *ccw* counterclockwise), which are associated with rotatory vertigo and oscillopsia. (b) Eye rotation axes (calculated from vector analysis of the pressure-induced eye movements) from behind (*left*), from above onto the head (*middle*), and from the right side (*right*) (reproduced with permission from Strupp et al. (2000))

Fig. 2.16 Schematic drawing of the
slow eye movements triggered by
stimulation of the left anterior
(superior) semicircular canal (*top*).
Eye movements result with a vertical
upward and (from the viewpoint of the
observer) torsional and
counterclockwise direction. *Bottom*:
the left labyrinth and the rotation axis
of the eyes calculated from the
three-dimensional vector analysis of
the pressure-induced eye movements
(see Fig. 2.15). The axis is
perpendicular to the plane of the
left anterior canal. *HC, AC, PC*
horizontal, superior, and posterior
semicircular canal

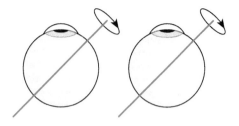

Eye movements

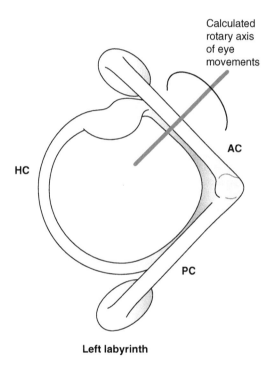

Left labyrinth

to a "third mobile window" (in addition to the round and oval windows in the
middle ear), which results in a pathological transmission of intracranial pressure changes to the perilymphatic space of the superior canal and thus causes
a stimulation/inhibition of the canal (due to ampullofugal or ampullopetal deviation of the cupula; Chien et al. 2011). Pressure is transmitted in the opposite
direction when sound triggers the attacks (Tullio phenomenon).

- A pathological mobility of the membrane of the oval or round window or the
  ossicular chain with a hypermobility of the stapes footplate (Dieterich et al.
  1989).
- A congenitally pathological bulging/prominence of the oval window causing a
  trans-stapedial CSF fistula, which leads to a perilymph hydrops and sensorineural
  hearing loss in children (Ehmer et al. 2010).

- Congenital anomalies of the inner ear such as Mondini malformation, which is often connected with an incomplete formation of the stapes footplate.
- Microfissures that spread from the ampulla of the posterior labyrinth to the round window.
- Bony defects in the region of the lateral wall of the labyrinth (toward the middle ear) together with a partial collapse of the perilymphatic space ("floating labyrinth"; Nomura et al. 1992) or in connection with a chronic otitis media, which can be associated with a dehiscence of the horizontal canal (Chien et al. 2011). Both lead to pathologically transmitted pressure from the middle ear to the labyrinth, for example, during a Valsalva maneuver.

The therapeutic principles derive from the pathophysiology: conservative (spontaneous) or operative closure of the fistula.

2.7.4 Pragmatic Therapy

The therapy of first choice for perilymph fistulas is conservative, as most fistulas close spontaneously.

Conservative therapy consists of 1–3 weeks of bed rest with moderate elevation of the head, if necessary a mild sedative, the administration of laxatives (to avoid pressing during bowel movements), and several weeks of limited physical activity that avoids all heavy lifting, abdominal pressing, strong coughing, or sneezing, even after improvement. This almost always leads to complete recovery (Singleton 1986). If conservative therapy fails and disturbing vestibular symptoms persist, exploratory tympanoscopy is indicated in order to examine the oval and round windows.

Surgical closure of the fistula successfully relieves vestibular vertigo in only up to 70 % of patients; the preexisting hearing loss generally does not improve at all. The operative procedure involves the removal of the mucous membrane in the region of the fistula and its substitution with autologous material (perichondral tissue of the tragus or fascia by means of gel foam). Fistulas in the oval window adjacent to the stapes footplate require a stapedectomy and prosthesis. Even if the operation is successful, the postoperative sensitivity of the patients to extreme physical strain (abdominal pressing, barotrauma) is greater than that of healthy subjects. Consequently, relapses occur not infrequently.

It is possible that a part of the fistulas that were earlier assumed to be in the middle ear were actually a dehiscence of the superior semicircular canal, as these can indirectly also lead to a pathological motility of the middle-ear window. This probably explains in part the low rate of improvement after the above-mentioned operations.

The *superior semicircular canal dehiscence syndrome* can be treated neurosurgically by covering the bony defect or by occlusion (the so-called plugging) of the canal (Minor 2005; Minor et al. 2001; Strupp et al. 2000). Prospective studies to determine which procedure is more effective are, however, still lacking. In a retrospective study involving 65 patients with the superior canal dehiscence syndrome, 20 patients had persisting disturbing symptoms. They underwent an operative treatment

(Minor 2005). In the course of the study, eight of nine patients with canal occlusion became symptom-free, whereas only 7 of 11 patients with coverage of the bony defect became free of symptoms, since four had a relapse after 3–6 months. Postoperative investigations indicate that there is some sensorineural hearing loss (Ward et al. 2012).

Double-sided occlusion of the superior canal was performed in cases of bilateral dehiscence syndrome. Although a few of these patients complained particularly of oscillopsia, they were apparently satisfied with the improvement of the other symptoms (Agrawal et al. 2012).

2.7.5 Differential Diagnosis and Clinical Problems

The differential diagnosis of perilymph fistulas includes the following illnesses:

- BPPV
- Central positioning/positional vertigo
- Menière's disease
- Vestibular paroxysmia
- Phobic postural vertigo
- Labyrinthine concussion
- Bilateral vestibulopathy

The presence of a perilymph fistula should be considered particularly in children who present with episodic vertigo with or without hearing loss and in patients who complain of vertigo and/or hearing loss after trauma of the ear or skull or barotrauma.

References

Adams ME, Kileny PR, Telian SA, El-Kashlan HK, Heidenreich KD, Mannrelli GR, et al. Electrocochlography as a diagnostic and intraoperative adjunct in superior semicircular canal dehiscence syndrome. Otol Neurotol. 2011;33:1506–12.

Agrawal Y, Minor LB, Schubert MC, Janky KL, Davalos-Bichara M, Carey JP. Second side surgery in superior canal dehiscence syndrome. Otol Neurotol. 2012;33:72–7.

Arbusow V, Strupp M, Dieterich M, Jäger L, Hischa A, Schulz P, et al. Alternating episodes of vestibular nerve excitation and failure. Neurology. 1998a;51:1480–3.

Arbusow V, Strupp M, Dieterich M, Stocker W, Naumann A, Schulz P, et al. Serum antibodies against membranous labyrinth in patients with "idiopathic" bilateral vestibulopathy. J Neurol. 1998b;245:132–6.

Arbusow V, Schulz P, Strupp M, Dieterich M, von Reinhardstoettner A, Rauch E, et al. Distribution of herpes simplex virus type 1 in human geniculate and vestibular ganglia: implications for vestibular neuritis. Ann Neurol. 1999;46:416–9.

Arbusow V, Theil D, Strupp M, Mascolo A, Brandt T. HSV-1 not only in human vestibular ganglia but also in the vestibular labyrinth. Audiol Neurootol. 2000;6:259–62.

Arbusow V, Theil D, Schulz P, Strupp M, Dieterich M, Rauch E, et al. Distribution of HSV-1 in human geniculate and vestibular ganglia: implications for vestibular neuritis. Ann N Y Acad Sci. 2003;1004:409–13.

Arbusow V, Derfuss T, Held K, Himmelein S, Strupp M, Gurkov R, et al. Latency of herpes simplex virus type-1 in human geniculate and vestibular ganglia is associated with infiltration of CD8+ T cells. J Med Virol. 2010;82:1917–20.

Ariyasu L, Byl FM, Sprague MS, Adour KK. The beneficial effect of methylprednisolone in acute vestibular vertigo. Arch Otolaryngol Head Neck Surg. 1990;116:700–3.

Asprella LG. Diagnostic and treatment strategy of lateral semicircular canal canalolithiasis. Acta Otorhinolaryngol Ital. 2005;25:277–83.

Bachmann-Harilstad G, Stenklev NC, Myrvoll E, Jablonski G, Klingenberg O. B-trace protein as a diagnostic marker for perilymphatic fluid fistula: a prospective controlled pilot study to test a sample collection technique. Otol Neurotol. 2011;32:7–10.

Baloh RW. Clinical practice. Vestibular neuritis. N Engl J Med. 2003;348:1027–32.

Baloh RW, Jacobson K, Winder T. Drop attacks with Meniere's syndrome. Ann Neurol. 1990; 28:384–7.

Baloh RW, Jacobsen K, Honrubia V. Horizontal semicircular canal variant of benign positional vertigo. Neurology. 1993;43:2542–9.

Baloh RW, Ishyama A, Wackym PA, Honrubia V. Vestibular neuritis: clinical-pathologic correlation. Otolaryngol Head Neck Surg. 1996;114:586–92.

Barrs DM. Intratympanic injections of dexamethasone for long-term control of vertigo. Laryngoscope. 2004;114:1910–4.

Battista RA. Audiometric findings of patients with migraine-associated dizziness. Otol Neurotol. 2004;25:987–92.

Bisdorff AR, Debatisse D. Localizing signs in positional vertigo due to lateral canal cupulolithiasis. Neurology. 2001;57:1085–8.

Brandt T. Vertigo; its multisensory syndromes. 2nd ed. Heidelberg/London/New York: Springer; 1999.

Brandt T, Daroff RB. Physical therapy for benign paroxysmal positional vertigo. Arch Otolaryngol. 1980;106:484–5.

Brandt T, Dieterich M. Vestibular paroxysmia: vascular compression of the eighth nerve? Lancet. 1994;343:798–9.

Brandt T, Steddin S. Current view of the mechanism of benign paroxysmal positioning vertigo: cupulolithiasis or canalolithiasis? J Vestib Res. 1993;3:373–82.

Brandt T, Steddin S, Daroff RB. Therapy for benign paroxysmal positioning vertigo, revisited. Neurology. 1994;44:796–800.

Brandt T, Strupp M, Arbusow V, Dieringer N. Plasticity of the vestibular system: central compensation and sensory substitution for vestibular deficits. Adv Neurol. 1997;73:297–309.

Brandt T, Schautzer F, Hamilton D, Brüning R, Markowitsch HJ, Kalla R, et al. Vestibular loss causes hippocampal atrophy and impaired spatial memory in humans. Brain. 2005;128:2732–41.

Brandt T, Huppert D, Hecht J, Karch C, Strupp M. Benign paroxysmal positioning vertigo: a long-term follow-up (6–17 years) of 125 patients. Acta Otolaryngol. 2006;126:160–3.

Brandt T, Huppert T, Hüfner K, Zingler VC, Dieterich M, Strupp M. Long-term course and relapses of vestibular and balance disorders. Restor Neurol Neurosci. 2010;28:69–82.

Büchele W, Brandt T. Vestibular neuritis – a horizontal semicircular canal paresis? Adv Otorhinolaryngol. 1988;42:157–61.

Büttner U, Helmchen C, Brandt T. Diagnostic criteria for central versus peripheral positioning nystagmus and vertigo: a review. Acta Otolaryngol. 1999;119:1–5.

Carey JP, Hirvonen T, Peng GC, Della-Santina CC, Cremer PD, Haslwanter T, et al. Changes in the angular vestibulo-ocular reflex after a single dose of intratympanic gentamicin for Meniere's disease. Auris Nasus Larynx. 2002;956:581–4.

Casani AP, Vannucci G, Fattori B, Berrettini S. The treatment of horizontal canal positional vertigo: our experience in 66 cases. Laryngoscope. 2002;112:172–8.

Casani AP, Piaggi P, Cerchiai N, Seccia V, Franceschini SS, Dallan I. Intratympanic treatment of intractable unilateral Meniere disease: gentamicin or dexamethasone? A randomized controlled trial. Otolaryngol Head Neck Surg. 2012;146:430–7.

Cawthorne T. The physiological basis for head exercises. J Chart Soc Physiother. 1944;30:106–7.

Cha YH, Brodsky J, Ishiyama G, Sabatti C, Baloh RW. The relevance of migraine in patients with Meniere's disease. Acta Otolaryngol. 2007;127:1241–5.

Chien WW, Carey JP, Minor LB. Canal dehiscence. Curr Opin Neurol. 2011;24:25–31.

Choung YH, Park K, Kim CH, Kim HJ, Kim K. Rare cases of Meniere's disease in children. J Laryngol Otol. 2006;120:343–52.

Claes J, Van-de-Heyning PH. Medical treatment of Meniere's disease: a review of literature. Acta Otolaryngol Suppl. 1997;526:37–42.

Cnyrim CD, Newman-Toker D, Karch C, Brandt T, Strupp M. Bedside differentiation of vestibular neuritis from central "vestibular pseudoneuritis". J Neurol Neurosurg Psychiatry. 2008;79: 458–60.

Cohen HS, Jerabek J. Efficacy of treatments for posterior canal benign paroxysmal positional vertigo. Laryngoscope. 1999;109:584–90.

Cohen HS, Kimball KT. Treatment variations on the Epley maneuver for benign paroxysmal positional vertigo. Am J Otolaryngol. 2004;25:33–7.

Cohen-Kerem R, Kisilevsky V, Einarson TR, Kozer E, Koren G, Rutka JA. Intratympanic gentamicin for Meniere's disease: a meta-analysis. Laryngoscope. 2004;114:2085–91.

Colletti V, Carner M, Colletti L. Auditory results after vestibular nerve section and intratympanic gentamicin for Meniere's disease. Otol Neurotol. 2007;28:145–51.

Coppo GF, Singarelli S, Fracchia P. Benign paroxysmal positional vertigo: follow-up of 165 cases treated by Semont's liberating maneuver. Acta Otorhinolaryngol Ital. 1996;16: 508–12.

De Stefano A, Dispenza F, De Donato G, Caruso A, Taibah A, Sanna M. Intratympanic gentamicin: a 1-day protocol treatment for unilateral Meniere's disease. Am J Otolaryngol. 2007;28: 289–93.

De Valck CF, Claes GM, Wuyts FL, Van de Heyning PH. Lack of diagnostic value of high-pass noise masking of auditory brainstem responses in Meniere's disease. Otol Neurotol. 2007;28: 700–7.

Deutschländer A, Glaser M, Strupp M, Dieterich M, Brandt T. Steroid treatment in bilateral vestibulopathy with inner ear antibodies. Acta Otolaryngol (Stockh). 2005;125:848–51.

Dieterich M, Brandt T, Fries W. Otolith function in man: results from a case of otolith Tullio phenomenon. Brain. 1989;112:1377–92.

Dieterich M, Bauermann T, Best C, Stoeter P, Schlindwein P. Evidence for cortical visual substitution of chronic bilateral vestibular failure (an fMRI study). Brain. 2007;130:2108–16.

Dutia MB. Mechanisms of vestibular compensation: recent advances. Curr Opin Otolaryngol Head Neck Surg. 2010;18:420–4.

Dziadziola JK, Laurikainen EL, Rachel JD, Quirk WS. Betahistine increases vestibular blood flow. Otolaryngol Head Neck Surg. 1999;120:400–5.

Ehmer DR, Booth T, Kutz JW, Roland PS. Radiographic diagnosis of trans-stapedial cerebrospinal fluid fistula. Otolaryngol Head Neck Surg. 2010;142(5):694–8.

Epley JM. The canalith repositioning procedure: for treatment of benign paroxysmal positional vertigo. Otolaryngol Head Neck Surg. 1992;107:399–404.

Fetter M, Dichgans J. Vestibular neuritis spares the inferior division of the vestibular nerve. Brain. 1996;119:755–63.

Fife TD, Iverson DJ, Lempert T, Furmann JM, Baloh RW, Tusa RJ, et al. Practice parameter: therapies for benign paroxysmal positional vertigo (an evidence-based review): report of the Quality Standards Subcommittee of the American Academy of Neurology. Neurology. 2008;70: 2067–74.

Fishman JM, Burgess C, Waddell A. Corticosteroids for the treatment of idiopathic acute vestibular dysfunction (vestibular neuritis). Cochrane Database Syst Rev. 2011;(5):CD008607.

Flanagan S, Mukherjee P, Tonkin J. Outcomes in the use of intra-tympanic gentamicin in the treatment of Meniere's disease. J Laryngol Otol. 2006;120:98–102.

Froehling DA, Bowen JM, Mohr DN, Brey RH, Beatty CW, Wollan PC, et al. The canalith repositioning procedure for the treatment of benign paroxysmal positional vertigo: a randomized controlled trial. Mayo Clin Proc. 2000;75:695–700.

Frykholm C, Larsen HC, Dahl N, Klar J, Rask-Andersen H, Friberg U. Familial Meniere's disease in five generations. Otol Neurotol. 2006;27:681–6.

Fujimoto C, Murofushi T, Chihara Y, Suzuki M, Yamasoba T, Iwasaki S. Novel subtype of idiopathic bilateral vestibulopathy: bilateral absence of vestibular evoked myogenic potentials in the presence of normal caloric responses. J Neurol. 2009;256:1488–92.

Gacek RR, Gacek MR. The three faces of vestibular ganglionitis. Ann Otol Rhinol Laryngol. 2002;111:103–14.

Garduno-Anaya MA, De Couthino TH, Hinojosa-Gonzalez R, Pane-Pianese C, Rios-Castaneda LC. Dexamethasone inner ear perfusion by intratympanic injection in unilateral Meniere's disease: a two-year prospective, placebo-controlled, double-blind, randomized trial. Otolaryngol Head Neck Surg. 2005;133:285–94.

Gates P. Hypothesis: could Meniere's disease be a channelopathy? Intern Med J. 2005;35:488–9.

Gianoli G, Goebel J, Mowry S, Poomipannit P. Anatomic differences in the lateral vestibular nerve channels and their implications in vestibular neuritis. Otol Neurotol. 2005;26:489–94.

Gordon CR, Gadoth N. Repeated vs single physical maneuver in benign paroxysmal positional vertigo. Acta Neurol Scand. 2004;110:166–9.

Goudakos JK, Markou KD, Franco-Vidal V, Vital V, Tsaligopoulos M, Darrouzet V. Corticosteroids in the treatment of vestibular neuritis: a systematic review and meta-analysis. Otol Neurotol. 2010;31:183–9.

Gufoni M, Mastrosimone L, Di Nasso F. Repositioning maneuver in benign paroxysmal vertigo of horizontal semicircular canal. Acta Otorhinolaryngol Ital. 1998;18:363–7.

Guinand N, Boselie F, Guyot JP, Kingma H. Quality of life of patients with bilateral vestibulopathy. Ann Otol Rhinol Laryngol. 2012;121:471–7.

Gürkov R, Flatz W, Louza J, Strupp M, Ertl-Wagner B, Krause E. In vivo visualized endolymphatic hydrops and inner ear function in patients with electrocochleographically confirmed Mèniere's disease. Otol Neurotol. 2012;33:1040–5.

Hain TC, Helminski JO, Reis IL, Uddin MK. Vibration does not improve results of the canalith repositioning procedure. Arch Otolaryngol Head Neck Surg. 2000;126:617–22.

Halmagyi GM, Curthoys IS. A clinical sign of canal paresis. Arch Neurol. 1988;45:737–9.

Hamann KF. Rehabilitation of patients with vestibular disorders. HNO. 1988;36:305–7.

Herdman SJ. Vestibular rehabilitation. Philadelphia: F.A. Davis Company; 2007.

Herdman SJ, Tusa RJ. Complications of the canalith repositioning procedure. Arch Otolaryngol Head Neck Surg. 1996;122:281–6.

Hillier SL, McDonnell M. Vestibular rehabilitation for unilateral peripheral vestibular dysfunction. Cochrane Database Syst Rev. 2011;(2):CD005397.

Hüfner K, Hamilton DA, Kalla R, Stephan T, Glasauer S, Ma J, et al. Spatial memory and hippocampal volume in humans with unilateral vestibular deafferentation. Hippocampus. 2007;17:471–85.

Hüfner K, Barresi D, Glaser M, Linn J, Adrion C, Mansmann U, et al. Vestibular paroxysmia: diagnostic features and medical treatment. Neurology. 2008a;71:1006–14.

Hüfner K, Linn J, Strupp M. Recurrent attacks of vertigo with monocular oscillopsia. Neurology. 2008b;71:863.

Hüfner K, Jahn K, Linn J, Strupp M, Brandt T. Vestibularisparoxysmie. Nervenheilkunde. 2009; 28:26–30.

Huppert D, Strupp M, Theil D, Glaser M, Brandt T. Low recurrence rate of vestibular neuritis: a long-term follow-up. Neurology. 2006;67:1870–1.

Huppert D, Strupp M, Brandt T. Long-term course of Meniere's disease revisited. Acta Otolaryngol. 2010;130:644–51.

Ihler F, Bertlich M, Sharaf K, Strieth S, Strupp M, Canis M. Betahistine exerts a dose-dependent effect on cochlear stria vascularis blood flow in Guinea pigs in vivo. PLoS One. 2012;7: e39086.

Ikezono T, Shindo S, Sekiguchi S, Moizane T, Pawankar R, Watanabe A, et al. The performance of Chochlin-tomoprotein detection test in the diagnosis of perilymphatic fistula. Audiol Neurootol. 2010;15:168–74.

Imai T, Ito M, Takeda N, Uno A, Matsunaga T, Sekine K, et al. Natural course of the remission of vertigo in patients with benign paroxysmal positional vertigo. Neurology. 2005;64:920–1.

Imai T, Takeda N, Ito M, Nakamae K, Sakae H, Fujioka H, et al. Three-dimensional analysis of benign paroxysmal positional nystagmus in a patient with anterior semicircular canal variant. Otol Neurotol. 2006;27:362–6.

Ishiyama G, Lopez IA, Ishiyama A. Aquaporins and Meniere's disease. Curr Opin Otolaryngol Head Neck Surg. 2006;14:332–6.

Ishiyama G, Lopez I, Baloh RW, Ishiyama A. Histopathology of the vestibular end organs after intratympanic gentamicin failure for Meniere's disease. Acta Otolaryngol. 2007;127:34–40.

James A, Thorp M. Meniere's disease. Clin Evid. 2005;(14):659–65.

Jannetta PJ, Møller MB, Møller AR. Disabling positional vertigo. N Engl J Med. 1984;310:1700–5.

Jeong SH, Choi SH, Kim JY, Koo JW, Kim HJ, Kim JS. Osteopenia and osteoporosis in idiopathic benign positional vertigo. Neurology. 2009;72:1069–76.

Jeong SH, Kim JS, Shin JW, Kim S, Lee H, Lee AY, et al. Decreased serum vitamin D in idiopathic benign paroxysmal positional vertigo. J Neurol. 2013;260(3):832–8.

Karlberg ML, Magnusson M. Treatment of acute vestibular neuronitis with glucocorticoids. Otol Neurotol. 2011;32:1140–3.

Karlberg M, Hall K, Quickert N, Hinson J, Halmagyi GM. What inner ear diseases cause benign paroxysmal positional vertigo? Acta Otolaryngol. 2000;120:380–5.

Kattah JC, Talkad AV, Wang DZ, Hsieh YH, Newman-Toker DE. HINTS to diagnose stroke in the acute vestibular syndrome: three-step bedside oculomotor examination more sensitive than early MRI diffusion-weighted imaging. Stroke. 2009;40:3504–10.

Kim JS, Kim HJ. Inferior vestibular neuritis. J Neurol. 2012;259:1553–60.

Kim HA, Lee H. Recent advances in central acute vestibular syndrome of a vascular cause. J Neurol Sci. 2012;321:17–22.

Kim YH, Kim KS, Kim KJ, Choi H, Choi JS, Hwang IK. Recurrence of vertigo in patients with vestibular neuritis. Acta Otolaryngol. 2011a;131:1172–7.

Kim S, Oh YM, Koo JW, Kim JS. Bilateral vestibulopathy: clinical characteristics and diagnostic criteria. Otol Neurotol. 2011b;32:812–7.

Kim JS, Oh SY, Lee SH, Kang JH, Kim DU, Jeong SH, et al. Randomized clinical trial for geotropic horizontal canal benign paroxysmal positional vertigo. Neurology. 2012a;79:700–7.

Kim JS, Oh SY, Lee SH, Kang JH, Kim DU, Jeong SH, et al. Randomized clinical trial for apogeotropic horizontal canal benign paroxysmal positional vertigo. Neurology. 2012b;78:159–66.

Kirchner H, Kremmyda O, Hüfner K, Stephan T, Zingler V, Brandt T, et al. Clinical, electrophysiological, and MRI findings in patients with cerebellar ataxia and a bilaterally pathological head-impulse test. Ann N Y Acad Sci. 2011;1233:127–38.

Klar J, Frykholm C, Friberg U, Dahl N. A Meniere's disease gene linked to chromosome 12p12.3. Am J Med Genet B Neuropsychiatr Genet. 2006;141:463–7.

Klockars T, Kentala E. Inheritance of Meniere's disease in the Finnish population. Arch Otolaryngol Head Neck Surg. 2007;133:73–7.

Lang J. Anatomy, length and blood vessel relations of "central" and "peripheral" paths of intracisternal cranial nerves. Zentralbl Neurochir. 1982;43:217–58.

Lange G, Maurer J, Mann W. Long-term results after interval therapy with intratympanic gentamicin for Meniere's disease. Laryngoscope. 2004;114:102–5.

Leal PR, Roch JA, Hermier M, Sonza MA, Caristino-Filho G, Sindou M. Structural abnormalities of the trigeminal root revealed by diffusion tensor imaging in patients with trigeminal neuralgia caused by neurovascular compression: a prospective, double-blind, controlled study. Pain. 2011;152:2357–64.

Lee H, Kim BK, Park HJ, et al. Prodromal dizziness in vestibular neuritis: frequency and clinical implication. J Neurol Neurosurg Psychiatry. 2009;80:355–6.

Lee GS, Zhou G, Poe D, Kenna M, Amin M, Ohlms L, et al. Clinical experience in diagnosis and management of superior semicircular dehiscence in children. Laryngoscope. 2011;121:2256–61.

Lempert T, Tiel-Wilck K. A positional maneuver for treatment of horizontal-canal benign positional vertigo. Laryngoscope. 1996;106:476–8.

Levrat E, Van Melle G, Monnier P, Maire R. Efficacy of the Semont maneuver in benign paroxysmal positional vertigo. Arch Otolaryngol Head Neck Surg. 2003;129:629–33.

Lezius F, Adrion C, Mansmann U, Jahn K, Strupp M. High-dosage betahistine dihydrochloride between 288 and 480 mg/day in patients with severe Meniere's disease: a case series. Eur Arch Otorhinolaryngol. 2011;268:1237–40.

Li Y, Zeng C, Luo T. Paroxysmal dysarthria and ataxia in multiple sclerosis and corresponding magnetic resonance imaging findings. J Neurol. 2011;258:273–6.

Lopez-Escamez JA, Gamiz MJ, Finana MG, Perez AF, Canet IS. Position in bed is associated with left or right location in benign paroxysmal positional vertigo of the posterior semicircular canal. Am J Otolaryngol. 2002;23:263–6.

Lynn S, Pool A, Rose D, Brey R, Suman V. Randomized trial of the canalith repositioning procedure. Otolaryngol Head Neck Surg. 1995;113:712–20.

MacDougall HG, Weber KP, McGarvie LA, Halmagyi GM, Curthoys IS. The video head impulse test: diagnostic accuracy in peripheral vestibulopathy. Neurology. 2009;73:1134–41.

Macias JD, Ellensohn A, Massingale S, Gerkin R. Vibration with the canalith repositioning maneuver: a prospective randomized study to determine efficacy. Laryngoscope. 2004;114:1011–4.

Magnusson M, Padoan S. Delayed onset of ototoxic effects of gentamicin in treatment of Meniere's disease. Rationale for extremely low dose therapy. Acta Otolaryngol (Stockh). 1991;111: 671–6.

Mandala M, Santoro GP, Libonati G, Casani AP, Faralli M, Giannoni B, et al. Double-blind randomized trial on short-term efficacy of the Semont maneuver for the treatment of posterior canal benign paroxysmal positional vertigo. J Neurol. 2012;259:882–5.

Marciano E, Marcelli V. Postural restrictions in labyrintholithiasis. Eur Arch Otorhinolaryngol. 2000;259:262–5.

Massoud EA, Ireland DJ. Post-treatment instructions in the nonsurgical management of benign paroxysmal positional vertigo. J Otolaryngol. 1996;25:121–5.

McClure JA. Horizontal canal BPV. J Otolaryngol. 1985;14:30–5.

Merchant SN, Adams JC, Nadol Jr JB. Pathophysiology of Meniere's syndrome: are symptoms caused by endolymphatic hydrops? Otol Neurotol. 2005;26:74–81.

Merfeld DM, Lewis RF. Replacing semicircular canal function with a vestibular implant. Curr Opin Otolaryngol Head Neck Surg. 2012;20:386–92.

Migliaccio AA, Halmagyi GM, McGarvie LA, Cremer PD. Cerebellar ataxia with bilateral vestibulopathy: description of a syndrome and its characteristic clinical sign. Brain. 2004;127: 280–93.

Minor LB. Clinical manifestation of superior semicircular canal dehiscence. Laryngoscope. 2005;115(10):1717–27.

Minor LB, Solomon D, Zinreich JS, Zee DS. Sound- and/or pressure-induced vertigo due to bone dehiscence of the superior semicircular canal. Arch Otolaryngol Head Neck Surg. 1998;124: 249–58.

Minor LB, Cremer PD, Carey JP, Della-Santina CC, Streubel SO, Weg N. Symptoms and signs in superior canal dehiscence syndrome. Ann NY Acad Sci. 2001;942:259–73.

Minor LB, Schessel DA, Carey JP. Meniere's disease. Curr Opin Neurol. 2004;17:9–16.

Møller MB, Møller AR, Janetta PJ, Sekhar L. Diagnosis and surgical treatment of disabling positional vertigo. J Neurosurg. 1986;64:21–8.

Nabi S, Parnes LS. Bilateral Meniere's disease. Curr Opin Otolaryngol Head Neck Surg. 2009;17:356–62.

Nadol Jr JB. Vestibular neuritis. Otolaryngol Head Neck Surg. 1995;112:162–72.

Neuhauser HK. Epidemiology of vertigo. Curr Opin Neurol. 2007;20:40–6.

Newman-Toker DE, Kattah JC, Alvernia JE, Wang DZ. Normal head impulse test differentiates acute cerebellar strokes from vestibular neuritis. Neurology. 2008;70:2378–85.

Niesten ME, McKenna MI, Hermann BS, Grolman W, Lee DJ. Utility of cVEMPs in bilateral superior canal dehiscence syndrome. Laryngoscope. 2013;123(1):226–32.

Nomura Y, Okuno T, Hara M, Young YH. "Floating" labyrinth. Pathophysiology and treatment of perilymph fistula. Acta Otolaryngol (Stockh). 1992;112:186–91.

Nuti D, Agus G, Barbieri MT, Passali D. The management of horizontal-canal paroxysmal positional vertigo. Acta Otolaryngol. 1998;118:455–60.

Oh HJ, Kim JS, Han BI, Lim JG. Predicting a successful treatment in posterior canal benign paroxysmal positional vertigo. Neurology. 2007;68:1219–22.

Ohbayashi S, Oda M, Yamamoto M, Urano M, Harada K, Horikoshi H, et al. Recovery of the vestibular function after vestibular neuronitis. Acta Otolaryngol Suppl (Stockh). 1993;503: 31–4.

Okinaka Y, Sekitani T, Okazaki H, Miura M, Tahara T. Progress of caloric response of vestibular neuronitis. Acta Otolaryngol Suppl (Stockh). 1993;503:18–22.

Phillips JS, Westerberg B. Intratympanic steroids for Meniere's disease or syndrome. Cochrane Database Syst Rev. 2011;(7):CD008514.

Postema RJ, Kingma CM, Wit HP, Albers FW, Van Der Laan BF. Intratympanic gentamicin therapy for control of vertigo in unilateral Meniere's disease: a prospective, double-blind, randomized, placebo-controlled trial. Acta Otolaryngol. 2008;128:876–80.

Pothier DD, Rutka JA, Ranalli PJ. Double impairment: clinical identification of 33 cases of cerebellar ataxia with bilateral vestibulopathy. Otolaryngol Head Neck Surg. 2011;146:804–8.

Pullens B, van Benthem PP. Intratympanic gentamicin for Ménière's disease or syndrome. Cochrane Database Syst Rev. 2011;(3):CD008234.

Pullens B, Verschuur HP, van Benthem PP. Surgery for Meniere's disease. Cochrane Database Syst Rev. 2013;(2):CD005395.

Radtke A, Neuhauser H, von Brevern M, Lempert T. A modified Epley's procedure for self-treatment of benign paroxysmal positional vertigo. Neurology. 1999;53:1358–60.

Radtke A, Lempert T, Gresty MA, Brookes GB, Bronstein AM, Neuhauser H. Migraine and Meniere's disease: is there a link? Neurology. 2002;59:1700–4.

Radtke A, von Brevern M, Tiel-Wilck K, Mainz-Perchalla A, Neuhauser H, Lempert T. Self-treatment of benign paroxysmal positional vertigo: Semont maneuver vs Epley procedure. Neurology. 2004;63:150–2.

Roberts RA, Gans RE, DeBoodt JL, Lister JJ. Treatment of benign paroxysmal positional vertigo: necessity of postmaneuver patient restrictions. J Am Acad Audiol. 2005;16: 357–66.

Ruckenstein MJ, Shepard NT. The canalith repositioning procedure with and without mastoid oscillation for the treatment of benign paroxysmal positional vertigo. ORL J Otorhinolaryngol Relat Spec. 2007;69:295–8.

Russell D, Baloh RW. Gabapentin responsive audiovestibular paroxysmia. J Neurol Sci. 2009; 281:99–100.

Sajjadi H, Paparella MM. Meniere's disease. Lancet. 2008;372:406–14.

Salvinelli F, Casale M, Trivelli M, D'Ascanio L, Firrisi L, Lamanna F, et al. Benign paroxysmal positional vertigo: a comparative prospective study on the efficacy of Semont's maneuver and no treatment strategy. Clin Ther. 2003;154:7–11.

Savastano M, Guerrieri V, Marioni G. Evolution of audiometric pattern in Meniere's disease: long-term survey of 380 cases evaluated according to the 1995 guidelines of the American Academy of Otolaryngology-Head and Neck Surgery. J Otolaryngol. 2006;35: 26–9.

Schmid-Priscoveanu A, Bohmer A, Obzina H, Straumann D. Caloric and search-coil head-impulse testing in patients after vestibular neuritis. J Assoc Res Otolaryngol. 2001;2:72–8.

Schuknecht HF. Pathology of the ear. Philadelphia: Lea & Febinger; 1993.

Schuknecht HF, Kitamura K. Vestibular neuritis. Ann Otol. 1981;90 Suppl 78:1–19.

Schüler O, Strupp M, Arbusow V, Brandt T. A case of possible autoimmune bilateral vestibulopathy treated with steroids. J Neurol Neurosurg Psychiatry. 2003;74:825.

Sekitani T, Imate Y, Noguchi T, Inokuma T. Vestibular neuronitis: epidemiological survey by questionnaire in Japan. Acta Otolaryngol Suppl (Stockh). 1993;503:9–12.

Selimoglu E. Aminoglycoside-induced ototoxicity. Curr Pharm Res. 2007;13:119–26.

Selmani Z, Marttila T, Pyykko I. Incidence of virus infection as a cause of Meniere's disease or endolymphatic hydrops assessed by electrocochleography. Eur Arch Otorhinolaryngol. 2005;262:331–4.

Semaan MT, Alagramam KN, Megerian CA. The basic science of Meniere's disease and endolymphatic hydrops. Curr Opin Otolaryngol Head Neck Surg. 2005;13:301–7.

Semont A, Freyss G, Vitte E. Curing the BPPV with a liberatory maneuver. Adv Otorhinolaryngol. 1988;42:290–3.

Sequeira SM, Whiting BR, Shimony JS, Vo KD, Hullar TE. Accuracy of computed tomography detection of superior canal dehiscence. Otol Neurotol. 2011;32:1500–5.

Serafini G, Palmieri AM, Simoncelli C. Benign paroxysmal positional vertigo of posterior semicircular canal: results in 160 cases treated with Semont's maneuver. Ann Otol Rhinol Laryngol. 1996;105:770–5.

Singleton GT. Diagnosis and treatment of perilymph fistulas without hearing loss. Otolaryngol Head Neck Surg. 1986;94:426–9.

Smith PF. Vestibular-hippocampal interactions. Hippocampus. 1997;7:465–71.

Soto-Varela A, Bartual-Magro J, Santos-Perez S, Vclez-Regueiro M, Lechuga-Garcia R, Perez-Carro-Rios A, et al. Benign paroxysmal vertigo: a comparative prospective study of the efficacy of Brandt and Daroff exercises, Semont and Epley maneuver. Rev Laryngol Otol Rhinol (Bord). 2001;122: 179–83.

Stapleton E, Mills R. Clinical diagnosis of Meniere's disease: how useful are the American Academy of Otolaryngology Head and Neck Surgery Committee on Hearing and Equilibrium guidelines? J Laryngol Otol. 2008;122:773–9.

Steddin S, Brandt T. Horizontal canal benign paroxysmal positioning vertigo (h-BPPV): transition of canalolithiasis to cupulolithiasis. Ann Neurol. 1996;40:918–22.

Steenerson RL, Cronin GW. Comparison of the canalith repositioning procedure and vestibular habituation training in forty patients with benign paroxysmal positional vertigo. Otolaryngol Head Neck Surg. 1996;114:61–4.

Steenerson RL, Cronin GW, Marbach PM. Effectiveness of treatment techniques in 923 cases of benign paroxysmal positional vertigo. Laryngoscope. 2005;115:226–31.

Stokroos R, Kingma H. Selective vestibular ablation by intratympanic gentamicin in patients with unilateral active Meniere's disease: a prospective, double-blind, placebo-controlled, randomized clinical trial. Acta Otolaryngol. 2004;124:172–5.

Straube A, Büttner U, Brandt T. Recurrent attacks with skew deviation, torsional nystagmus, and contraction of the left frontalis muscle. Neurology. 1994;44:177–8.

Strupp M, Brandt T. Peripheral vestibular disorders. Curr Opin Neurol. 2013;26:81–9.

Strupp M, Brandt T, Steddin S. Horizontal canal benign paroxysmal positioning vertigo: reversible ipsilateral caloric hypoexcitability caused by canalolithiasis? Neurology. 1995;45:2072–6.

Strupp M, Arbusow V, Maag KP, Gall C, Brandt T. Vestibular exercises improve central vestibulospinal compensation after vestibular neuritis. Neurology. 1998;51:838–44.

Strupp M, Eggert T, Straube A, Jäger L, Querner V, Brandt T. "Innere Perilymphfistel" des anterioren Bogengangs. Nervenarzt. 2000;71:138–42.

Strupp M, Zingler VC, Arbusow V, Niklas D, Maag KP, Dieterich M, et al. Methylprednisolone, valacyclovir, or the combination for vestibular neuritis. N Engl J Med. 2004;351:354–61.

Strupp M, Cnyrim C, Brandt T. Vertigo and dizziness: treatment of benign paroxysmal positioning vertigo, vestibular neuritis and Menère's disease. In: Candelise L, editor. Evidence-based neurology – management of neurological disorders. Oxford: Blackwell Publishing; 2007. p. 59–69.

Strupp M, Huppert D, Frenzel C, Wagner J, Zingler VC, Mansmann U, et al. Long-term prophylactic treatment of attacks of vertigo in Menière's disease – comparison of a high with a low dosage of betahistine in an open trial. Acta Otolaryngol (Stockh). 2008;128:620–4.

Strupp M, Thurtell MJ, Shaikh AG, Brandt T, Zee DS, Leigh RJ. Pharmacotherapy of vestibular and ocular motor disorders, including nystagmus. J Neurol. 2011;258:1207–22.

Strupp M, Stuckrad-Barre S, Brandt T, Tonn JC. Compression of the eighth cranial nerve causes vestibular paroxysmia. Neurology 2013;80:e77.

Szmulewicz DJ, Waterston JA, Halmagyi GM, Mossman S, Chancellor AM, Mclean CA, et al. Sensory neuropathy as part of the cerebellar ataxia neuropathy vestibular areflexia syndrome. Neurology. 2011;76:1903–10.

Takumida M, Kakigi A, Takeda T, Anniko M. Meniere's disease: a long-term follow-up study of bilateral hearing levels. Acta Otolaryngol. 2006;126:921–5.

Thabet EM, Abdelkhalek A, Zghloul H. Superior semicircular canal dehiscence syndrome as assessed by oVEMP and temporal bone computed tomography imaging. Eur Arch Otorhinolaryngol. 2012;269:1545–9.

Theil D, Arbusow V, Derfuss T, Strupp M, Pfeiffer M, Mascolo A, et al. Prevalence of HSV-1 LAT in human trigeminal, geniculate, and vestibular ganglia and its implication for cranial nerve syndromes. Brain Pathol. 2001;11:408–13.

Thirlwall AS, Kundu S. Diuretics for Meniere's disease or syndrome. Cochrane Database Syst Rev. 2006;(3):CD003599.

van de Berg R, Guinand N, Guyot JP, Kingma H, Stokroos RJ. The modified ampullar approach for vestibular implant surgery: feasibility and its first application in a human with a long-term vestibular loss. Front Neurol. 2012;3:18.

Vannucchi P, Giannoni B, Pagnini P. Treatment of horizontal semicircular canal benign paroxysmal positional vertigo. J Vestib Res. 2000;7:1–6.

Vital D, Hegemann SC, Straumann D, Bergamin O, Bockisch CJ, Angehrn D, et al. A new dynamic visual acuity test to assess peripheral vestibular function. Arch Otolaryngol Head Neck Surg. 2010;136:686–91.

von Brevern M, Schmidt T, Schonfeld U, Lempert T, Clarke AH. Utricular dysfunction in patients with benign paroxysmal positional vertigo. Otol Neurotol. 2006a;27:92–6.

von Brevern M, Seelig T, Radtke A, Tiel-Wilck K, Neuhauser H, Lempert T. Short-term efficacy of Epley's manoeuvre: a double-blind randomised trial. J Neurol Neurosurg Psychiatry. 2006b;77:980–2.

von Brevern M, Radtke A, Lezius F, Feldmann M, Ziese T, Lempert T, et al. Epidemiology of benign paroxysmal positional vertigo: a population based study. J Neurol Neurosurg Psychiatry. 2007;78:710–5.

Wagner JN, Glaser M, Brandt T, Strupp M. Downbeat nystagmus: aetiology and comorbidity in 117 patients. J Neurol Neurosurg Psychiatry. 2008;79:672–7.

Ward BK, Agrawal Y, Nguyen E, Della Santina CC, Limb CI, Francis HW, et al. Hearing outcomes after surgical plugging of the superior semicircular canal by a middle fossa approach. Otol Neurotol. 2012;33:1386–91.

Watson SR, Halmagyi GM, Colebatch JG. Vestibular hypersensitivity to sound (Tullio phenomenon): structural and functional assessment. Neurology. 2000;54:722–8.

Woodworth BA, Gillespie MB, Lambert PR. The canalith repositioning procedure for benign positional vertigo: a meta-analysis. Laryngoscope. 2004;114:1143–6.

Yacovino DA, Hain TC, Gualtieri F. New therapeutic maneuver for anterior canal benign paroxysmal positional vertigo. J Neurol. 2009;256:1851–5.

Yeh TH, Herman P, Tsai MC, Tran-Ba-Huy P, Van-den-Abbeele T. A cationic nonselective stretch-activated channel in the Reissner's membrane of the guinea pig cochlea. Am J Physiol. 1998;274:C566–76.

Yimtae K, Srirompotong S, Sae-Seaw P. A randomized trial of the canalith repositioning procedure. Laryngoscope. 2003;113:828–32.

Zhang LC, Sha Y, Dai CF. Another etiology for vertigo due to idiopathic lateral semicircular canal bony defect. Auris Nasus Larynx. 2011;38:402–5.

Zingler VC, Cnyrim C, Jahn K, Weintz E, Fernbacher J, Frenzel C, et al. Causative factors and epidemiology of bilateral vestibulopathy in 255 patients. Ann Neurol. 2007a;61:524–32.

Zingler VC, Weintz E, Jahn K, Mike A, Huppert D, Rettinger N, et al. Follow-up of vestibular function in bilateral vestibulopathy. J Neurol Neurosurg Psychiatry. 2007b;79:284–8.

Zingler VC, Weintz E, Jahn K, Bötzel K, Wagner J, Huppert D, et al. Saccular function less affected than canal function in bilateral vestibulopathy. J Neurol. 2008;255:1332–6.

Chapter 3
Central Vestibular Forms of Vertigo

3.1 Central Vestibular Syndromes

The usual classification of vestibular disorders is based on the anatomical lesion site and distinguishes between the peripheral vestibular system and the central vestibular system. The first includes the labyrinth and the vestibular nerve, i.e., the first and second neurons. The latter involves central vestibular nuclei and pathways beginning in the vestibular nuclei at the level of the pontomedullary brainstem. Consequently, lacunar infarctions or MS plaques that affect the root entry zone of the eighth nerve are assigned to the central syndromes (central vestibular pseudoneuritis; see below); however, in a strict sense, they represent a peripheral disorder, since they affect the second afferent vestibular neuron. We would like to propose a third category, which is based on functional rather than anatomical characteristics, namely, disorders of higher vestibular function.

3.1.1 Disorders of Higher Vestibular Function

The term "disorders of higher visual function" is well established in neuro-ophthalmology. It usually correlates circumscribed supratentorial especially cortical lesions with particular dysfunctions of "higher visual perception," recognition and memory, as well as spatial orientation along the ventral and dorsal streams (Milner and Goodale 1995; Goodale 2011). Analogously one could also define disorders of higher vestibular function. These disorders are characterized by complex perceptual, sensorimotor, and behavioral criteria that exceed the basic perceptions like body motion and motor responses as well as the vestibulo-ocular and vestibulospinal reflexes. There are differences and similarities between these higher vestibular/visual disorders. A typical difference is that higher vestibular disorders often involve other sensory modalities, whereas higher visual disorders do not. Similarities are that both manifest with cognitive disturbances of spatial orientation, attention, spatial memory, and navigation. Sometimes, however, it is not possible to differentiate between them. This becomes evident in syndromes like visuospatial hemineglect (Karnath and Rorden 2012; Brandt et al. 2012) or the room-tilt illusion with transient episodes of "upside-down vision" induced by a vestibular tonus imbalance (Tiliket et al. 1996; Brandt 1997; Sierra-Hidalgo et al. 2012). Not all disorders of higher vestibular function are caused by lesions of central vestibular structures. Peripheral bilateral vestibular loss, for example, not only causes oscillopsia and postural imbalance due to insufficient vestibulo-ocular and vestibulospinal reflexes but also impairs spatial memory and navigation because of a lack of vestibular input to the hippocampal formation (Sect. 2.5).

In the following the focus is on central vestibular syndromes, some of which are disorders of higher vestibular function as defined above.

3.1.2 Central Vestibular Structures

Central vestibular forms of vertigo are caused by lesions along the vestibular pathways in the brainstem, which extend from the vestibular nuclei in the medulla oblongata to the ocular motor nuclei and integration centers in the rostral midbrain and to the vestibulocerebellum, the thalamus, and multisensory vestibular cortex areas in the temporoparietal cortex (Brandt and Dieterich 1995; Dieterich and Brandt 2008; Baier and and Dieterich 2009). These forms of vertigo are often clearly defined clinical syndromes of various etiologies, with typical

- ocular motor,
- perceptual, and
- postural manifestations

that permit a precise topographic diagnosis of brainstem lesions. The clinical examination of eye movements and of nystagmus is important for localizing the lesion site (Büttner et al. 1995; Büttner-Ennever 2008).

The most important structures of central vestibular forms of vertigo are the neuronal pathways mediating the vestibulo-ocular reflex (VOR). They travel from the peripheral labyrinth over the vestibular nuclei in the medullary brainstem to the ocular motor nuclei (III, IV, VI) and the supranuclear integration centers in the pons and midbrain (interstitial nucleus of Cajal, INC; and rostral interstitial nucleus of the medial longitudinal fascicle, riMLF) (Brandt and Dieterich 1994, 1995; Fig. 3.1). Compensatory eye movements are generated over this three-neuron reflex arc during rapid head and body movements. Additionally important are the interstitial nucleus of Cajal, the INC, and the rostral interstitial nucleus of the MLF, the riMLF, as integration centers in the midbrain for vertical and torsional eye movements, as well as the nucleus prepositus hypoglossi together with the vestibular nuclei and the cerebellum as integration centers for horizontal eye movements.

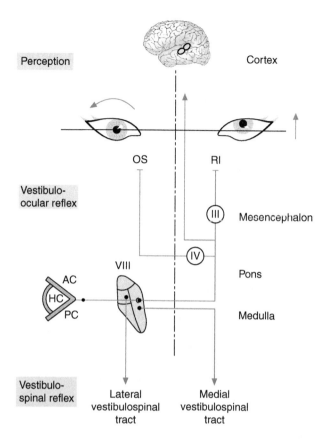

Fig. 3.1 Schematic drawing representing the vestibulo-ocular reflex (VOR) with its three-neuron reflex arc and its mediation of ocular motor, perceptual, and postural functions, as well as an ocular tilt reaction with ocular torsion and vertical divergence of the eyes due to a tonus imbalance of the graviceptive pathways. *AC* anterior semicircular canal, *HC* horizontal canal, *PC* posterior canal; *RI* inferior rectus muscle, *OS* superior oblique muscle; III, IV, VIII nuclei of cranial nerves

Ascending pathways travel both contralaterally and ipsilaterally over the posterolateral thalamus up to a network of vestibular areas in the parietotemporal cortex and the insula, e.g., the parietoinsular vestibular cortex (PIVC), and areas in the superior temporal gyrus and inferior parietal lobes, which are primarily responsible for perception, self-motion, and orientation in space. These cortical network areas—with the PIVC as a core region—all receive multisensory input. Parallel to the data of animal studies (Grüsser et al. 1990a, b; Chen et al. 2011), functional imaging in humans with MRI and PET allowed visualization of a similar cortical network activated by caloric irrigation or galvanic stimulation of the peripheral vestibular system (Brandt and Dieterich 1999; Dieterich and Brandt 2008) as well as its functional connectivity (zu Eulenburg et al. 2012). This network showed a dominance for vestibular cortical function lying in the nondominant hemisphere, i.e., in the right hemisphere in right-handers (Dieterich et al. 2003).

Descending pathways lead from the vestibular nuclei along the medial and lateral vestibulospinal tract into the spinal cord to mediate postural control. In addition, there are numerous pathways to the vestibulocerebellum.

Thus, disorders of the VOR are characterized not only by ocular motor deficits but also by disorders of perception (due to impaired vestibulocortical projections of the VOR) and by disorders of postural control (due to impaired vestibulospinal projections of the VOR) (Fig. 3.1).

Central vestibular syndromes are generally the result of lesions of these pathways or of core areas most often caused by:

- Infarction
- Hemorrhage
- Tumor
- Multiple sclerosis plaque
- Degenerative brain diseases.

Pathological stimulations as occur in paroxysmal brainstem attacks (with ataxia and dysarthria) in MS or lacunar infarctions are more seldom the cause. Vestibular epilepsy is even rarer. Table 3.1 provides an overview of ischemic lesions caused by lacunar or territorial infarctions in the region of the central vestibular system, giving the typical clinical syndromes and vascular territories.

3.1.3   Clinical Aspects, Course of Disease, Pathophysiology, and Therapeutic Principles

As a rule unilateral lesions of the bilaterally organized central vestibular pathways cause vestibular syndromes as a consequence of a vestibular tonus imbalance. Surprisingly, acute unilateral lesions of the multiple vestibular cortex areas due to, e.g., a middle cerebral artery infarction, manifest without vestibular symptoms such as vertigo (Anagnostou et al. 2010). Only single cases have been described of patients with such strokes involving the vestibular cortex who presented with nonepileptic rotational vertigo, nystagmus, and postural imbalance, which gradually improved within days (Brandt et al. 1995; Naganuma et al. 2006). Vestibular epilepsy, i.e., epileptic vertigo, due to excitation of the temporo–parieto–occipital junction, is also a rare condition (Brandt 1999; Hewett et al. 2011).

There are two clinically relevant syndromes, the spatial hemineglect and the pusher syndrome, which occur with acute unilateral thalamic or hemispheric lesions.

Table 3.1 Clinical syndrome and corresponding arterial territory affected by unilateral vascular lesions

Brain site/clinical syndrome	Artery
Medulla oblongata	
Wallenberg's syndrome (DVD) with OTR and its features (head tilt, vertical divergence of the eyes, ocular torsion, deviation of the SVV) ipsiversive: lesion of the medial vestibular nuclei	Branches of the vertebral artery or PICA Rare: posterior spinal artery
"Vestibular pseudo-neuritis" (DVD)	Branches of the vertebral artery or PICA
OTR ipsiversive: lesion of the superior vestibular nuclei	Branches of the AICA
Pons and midbrain	
OTR or its components toward the opposite side: lesion of the MLF	Paramedian arteries of the basilar artery
UBN in combination with INO: lesion of the superior vestibular nuclei and the CVTT	Paramedian arteries from the basilar artery
SVV tilt ipsiversive: lesion of the medial lemniscus (IVTT)	Paramedian arteries from the basilar artery
Rostral midbrain	
OTR or its components contraversive: lesion of the INC and riMLF	Paramedian midbrain arteries from the basilar artery
Paramedian thalamus	
OTR contraversive to the lesion, only if rostral midbrain is affected (INC lesion)	50 % of the paramedian midbrain arteries originate with the paramedian thalamus arteries from the basilar artery
Posterolateral thalamus	
Tendency to fall to the side, SVV deviation, perhaps also astasia ipsiversive or contraversive	Thalamogeniculate arteries or perhaps branches of the posterior cerebral artery
Temporoparietal cortex	
Tendency to fall to the side, SVV deviation mainly contraversive, perhaps pusher syndrome	Branches of the middle cerebral artery
Vestibulocerebellum	
OTR with its components contraversive (ca. 60 %) or ipsiversive (ca. 25 %): lesions of the uvula/nodulus/dentate nucleus or parts of the cerebellar hemispheres	Branches of the PICA and AICA

OTR ocular tilt reaction, *MLF* medial longitudinal fascicle, *riMLF* rostral interstitial nucleus of the MLF, *INC* interstitial nucleus of Cajal, *CVTT* central ventral tegmental tract, *IVTT* ipsilateral vestibulothalamic tract, *SVV* subjective visual vertical, *AICA* anterior inferior cerebellar artery, *PICA* posterior inferior cerebellar artery

These conditions are not merely vestibular disorders; they reflect a dysfunction of spatial orientation, attention, and postural control—all based on multisensory integration (visual, vestibular, somatosensory). Both syndromes, however, have features that can best be explained by the dysfunction of the vestibular system, e.g., with the dominance of the right hemisphere in right-handers. These disorders of higher vestibular function involve not only convergence of multisensory input but also sensorimotor integration with spatial memory, orientation, attention, navigation, and the interaction of body and surrounding during locomotion.

In general, the beginning and duration of the symptoms help in the differential diagnosis of central vestibular forms of vertigo:

- Short rotatory or postural vertigo attacks lasting seconds to minutes or for a few hours are caused by transient ischemic attacks within the vertebrobasilar territory, vestibular migraine, paroxysmal brainstem attacks with ataxia/dysarthria in MS, and rarely by vestibular epilepsy.
- Attacks of rotatory or postural vertigo lasting hours to several days, generally with additional brainstem deficits, can be caused by an infarction, hemorrhage, or MS plaque in the brainstem, seldom by a long-lasting attack of vestibular migraine.
- Several days to weeks of persisting postural vertigo (seldom persisting rotatory vertigo), combined with a tendency to fall in a certain direction, is usually caused by permanent damage to the brainstem or the cerebellum bilaterally, e.g., downbeat nystagmus syndrome (http://extra.springer.com) due to permanently degenerative cerebellar disease or upbeat nystagmus syndrome (http://extra.springer.com) due to paramedian pontomedullary or pontomesencephalic damage (infarction, hemorrhage, tumor, intoxication).

3.1.4 Differential Diagnostics: Peripheral Versus Central Vertigo

In the acute phase following the sudden occurrence of rotatory or postural vertigo, the first question that arises concerns the differential diagnosis (see also p. 76): is it a peripheral or a central vestibular vertigo caused, for example, by an acute stroke? If it is, specific diagnostics and therapy must be begun without delay. Thus, if the main symptom is acute vertigo, the following 5-step procedure is recommended for the first examination:

1. Perform the head-impulse test (Cnyrim et al. 2008; Kattah et al. 2009; Newman-Toker et al. 2008).
2. Look for a skew deviation (vertical divergence) using the cover test (Fig. 1.4).
3. Look for peripheral vestibular spontaneous nystagmus (with Frenzel's glasses) as opposed to central fixation nystagmus (Fig. 1.10).
4. Look for a gaze-evoked nystagmus beating in the opposite direction of a possible spontaneous nystagmus or vertically upward/downward.
5. Look for deficits of smooth pursuit and saccades, especially in the vertical direction.

The presence of a skew deviation, a normal head-impulse test (Newman-Toker et al. 2008), and a gaze-evoked nystagmus in the opposite direction to that of spontaneous nystagmus in an acute vestibular syndrome indicates a lesion of the brainstem or, more seldom, a lesion of the cerebellum.

A stroke can be indicated even if the head-impulse test is pathological and thus suggests a peripheral labyrinthine disorder. The above-described 5-step procedure indicates the presence of central ischemia with a sensitivity of more than 90 %; this sensitivity is higher than that possible with an early MRI with diffusion-weighted sequences (88 %) (Kattah et al. 2009). It must be stressed that after an acute, isolated episode of vertigo, the risk of having a stroke in the next 4 years amounts to ca. 6 %. This is threefold higher than the risk in an age-matched control group; if there are additional vascular risk factors, then the risk is even 5.5-fold higher (Lee et al. 2011).

3.1.5 Central Vestibular Syndromes in the Three Planes of Action of the VOR

For a simple clinical overview, the central vestibular brainstem syndromes can be classified according to the three major planes of action of the VOR (Brandt and Dieterich 1994, 1995) (Figs. 3.2 and 3.3).

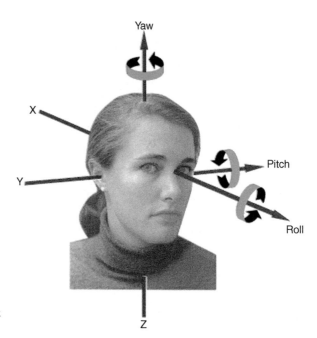

Fig. 3.2 Orientation of the three major planes of action of the vestibulo-ocular reflex (VOR): yaw, pitch, and roll

Fig. 3.3 Schematic drawing of the brainstem and cerebellum with the typical sites of lesions that induce vestibular syndromes in the three planes of the VOR; *III, IV, VI, VIII* cranial nerve nuclei; *MLF* medial longitudinal fascicle; *riMLF* rostral interstitial nucleus of the medial longitudinal fascicle; *INC* interstitial nucleus of Cajal

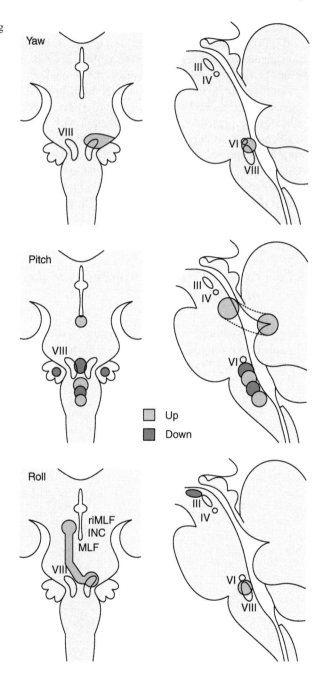

Overview 3.1 Syndromes of the VOR and Its Clinical Symptoms
Horizontal Plane (Yaw):
- "Vestibular pseudoneuritis" (http://extra.springer.com)
- Spontaneous horizontal nystagmus (fixation nystagmus)
- Horizontal past-pointing to the right/left ("subjective straight ahead")
- Postural instability
- Tendency to fall to one side
- Turning in the Unterberger stepping test

Sagittal Plane (Pitch):
- Downbeat/upbeat nystagmus (http://extra.springer.com)
- Deviation of the subjective horizontal upward or downward
- Past-pointing to up/down ("subjective straight ahead")
- Postural instability
- Tendency to fall forward or backward

Frontal Plane (Roll):
- Ocular tilt reaction (http://extra.springer.com) with
  Skew deviation
  Ocular torsion
  Head tilt and
  Deviation of the SVV
- Postural instability
- Tendency to fall to one side
- Pushing possible

3.1.5.1 Central Vestibular Syndromes in the Horizontal (Yaw) Plane

As far as we now know, central syndromes in yaw are caused only by lesions in the area of:

- The entry zone of the vestibular nerve into the medulla oblongata
- The medial vestibular nuclei
- The neighboring integration centers for horizontal eye movements (nucleus prepositus hypoglossi and paramedian pontine reticular formation, PPRF) (Figs. 3.3 and 3.4).

Other clinical signs are:

- Ipsilateral caloric hyporesponsiveness
- Horizontal gaze deviation
- A tendency to fall to the affected side (lateropulsion)
- Past-pointing, corresponding to a deviation of the "subjective straight ahead".

The clinical symptoms are similar to those of an acute peripheral vestibular lesion as occurs in vestibular neuritis and thus is also called "vestibular pseudoneuritis." A purely central yaw plane syndrome is rare because the area of a lesion that can theoretically cause a pure tonus imbalance in the yaw plane adjoins and in part

Fig. 3.4 Magnetic resonance image of a patient with "vestibular pseudoneuritis," a disorder of the vestibulo-ocular reflex (VOR) in the yaw plane. In the T2-weighted sequence there is a visible pontomedullary brainstem MS lesion on the right side, which impairs the fascicle of the eighth cranial nerve

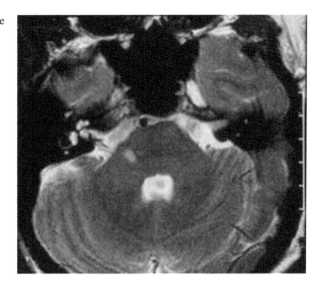

overlaps with structures in the vestibular nuclei, which are also responsible for vestibular function in the roll plane. Thus, skew deviation is the only specific but not very sensitive sign that indicates a pseudo-vestibular neuritis as opposed to vestibular neuritis (Cnyrim et al. 2008). The horizontal head-impulse test also does not allow a clear differentiation between neuritis and pseudoneuritis: 9 % of patients with a pontocerebellar infarction have a pathological head-impulse test as well (Newman-Toker et al. 2008).

A normal head-impulse test in a patient with an acute vestibular syndrome and nystagmus indicates in practically all cases a central lesion (Newman-Toker et al. 2008).

The most common causes include MS plaques or ischemic infarctions within the area of the vestibular nuclei or fascicles (Brandt et al. 1986; Hopf 1987; Kim and Lee 2010). If the lesion extends beyond the vestibular nuclei, other accompanying brainstem symptoms can be detected. Since a unilateral medullary ischemic or inflammatory brainstem lesion is as a rule present, the prognosis is favorable because central compensation takes place over the opposite side. The symptoms can be expected to resolve slowly—as in vestibular neuritis—within days to weeks (Dieterich and Brandt 1992; Cnyrim et al. 2007; Fig. 3.5). In such cases central compensation can be promoted by early balance training together with the simultaneous treatment of the underlying illness.

3.1.5.2   Central Vestibular Syndromes in the Sagittal (Pitch) Plane

Vestibular syndromes in the sagittal (pitch) plane have so far been attributed to lesions in the following sites:

- Paramedian bilaterally in the medullary and pontomedullary brainstem
- The pontomesencephalic brainstem (with the adjacent cerebellar peduncle)

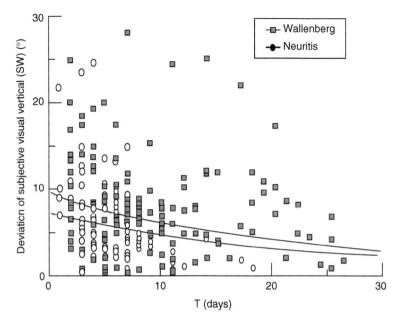

Fig. 3.5 The time course of SVV deviations in 50 patients with ischemic lesion in the vestibular nucleus (Wallenberg's syndrome) and 50 patients with vestibular neuritis shows that normalization takes place within about 4 weeks (Reproduced with permission from Cnyrim et al. (2007))

- In the paramedian pons
- The flocculus/paraflocculus of the cerebellum, bilaterally.

Despite the numerous clinical studies on upbeat (UBN) and downbeat (DBN) nystagmus as well as the many hypotheses proposed to explain their pathomechanism, so far the pathophysiology of these disorders has not been clarified (Halmagyi and Leigh 2004; Glasauer et al. 2003, 2005a, b; Marti et al. 2005; Pierrot-Deseilligny and Milea 2005). There seem to be various forms of DBN responsible for different aspects of the disorder. Several pathomechanisms that cause an instability in the brainstem–cerebellar networks, which normally stabilize vertical gaze, are currently being discussed, for example, an asymmetry:

- In the vertical neuronal integrator with a disorder of the saccade generator, which is conspicuous in eccentric gaze positions
- In the central connections of the VOR for vertical eye movements including the otolithic pathways, which explains the frequent dependence on gravity
- In the vertical gaze pursuit system with spontaneous upward drift.

Here the flocculus/paraflocculus seems to play a special role, since its damage leads to a disinhibition of the vestibular pathways of the superior vestibular nucleus to the oculomotor nucleus (Zee et al. 1981). This fits with findings from functional imaging studies which have proven that patients with idiopathic downbeat nystagmus have a hypometabolism or a reduced activity in the flocculus/paraflocculus as well as in the pontomedullary brainstem (Bense et al. 2006; Kalla et al. 2006; Hüfner et al. 2007; Figs. 3.6 and 3.7). In contrast, structural MRI found atrophies of the gray matter not in the flocculus/paraflocculus but in the lateral portions of the cerebellar hemispheres (lobule VI) and in the oculomotor vermis (Hüfner et al. 2007).

The dependence of the intensity of DBN on the head position suggests a disorder of the otolithic pathways in some cases (intensity is less in the upright position than in the prone or supine positions). Similarly, the efficacy of drug treatment with the potassium channel blocker 4-aminopyridine can depend on position (Spiegel et al. 2010; Sander et al. 2011).

Downbeat Nystagmus Syndrome (DBN)

The downbeat nystagmus syndrome (DBN) (http://extra.springer.com) is the most frequently acquired fixational nystagmus. It beats downward in primary gaze

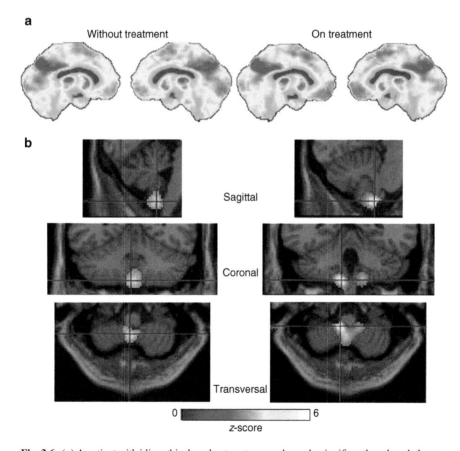

Fig. 3.6 (**a**) A patient with idiopathic downbeat nystagmus showed a significantly reduced glucose metabolism (FDG-PET) in the flocculus/paraflocculus (*left*), which improved as the clinical syndrome improved after administration of 4-aminopyridine (*right*) (reproduced with permission from Bense et al. (2006)). (**b**) A reduction of the activations in the flocculus (fMRI) was also observed in patients with downbeat nystagmus during vertical gaze pursuit movements (Reproduced with permission from Kalla et al. (2006))

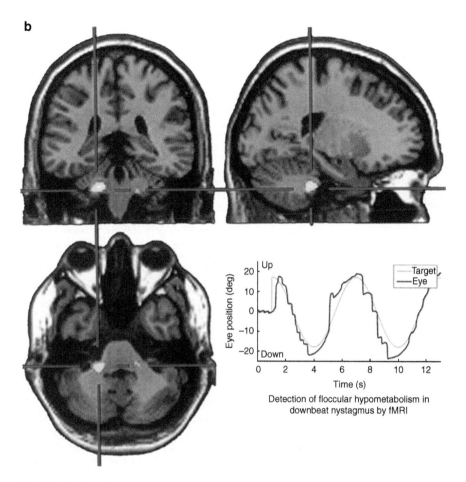

b

Eye position (deg)

Up
20
10
0
-10
-20
Down

Target
Eye

0 2 4 6 8 10 12

Time (s)

Detection of floccular hypometabolism in
downbeat nystagmus by fMRI

Fig. 3.6 (continued)

position, is exacerbated on lateral gaze and in head-hanging position, and can have a rotatory component. It is accompanied by a combination of visual and vestibulo-cerebellar ataxia with a:

- Tendency to fall backward
- Past-pointing upward (Dieterich et al. 1998)
- Disturbance of vertical gaze pursuit (Leigh and Zee 2006).

DBN is often associated with other ocular motor, cerebellar, and vestibular disorders, e.g., disorders of gaze pursuit, OKN, or the visual suppression of the VOR. The intensity of idiopathic DBN can be dependent on head position and on the time of day: it is stronger in the morning than at noon or in the afternoon (Spiegel et al. 2009). The syndrome is frequently persistent. DBN is often the result of a bilateral lesion of the flocculus or the paraflocculus (Kalla et al. 2006) (mainly

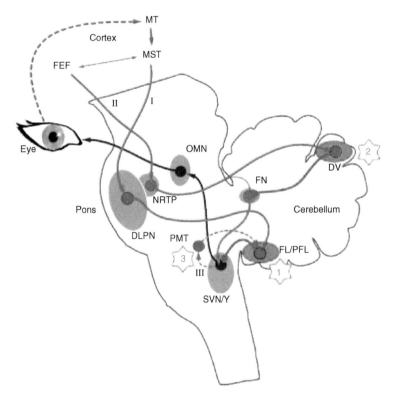

Fig. 3.7 Schematic drawing of a model of the pathomechanism of downbeat nystagmus. The model assumes a common final stretch for the pathways that cause the disinhibition of neurons of the superior vestibular nucleus and of the Y group (Reproduced with permission from Hüfner et al. (2007)). Oculomotor connections of the gaze pursuit system (I, II) and of the vertical gaze stabilization (III) are affected. Various lesion sites (1–3) can evoke downbeat nystagmus

atrophy of the cerebellum, rarely intoxication due to anticonvulsant drugs). It is more rarely induced by a lesion on the floor of the fourth ventricle (Leigh and Zee 2006). Accordingly idiopathic cases occur most often (38 %), degenerative disorders of the cerebellum in 20 % of cases, vascular lesions in 9 %, and malformations in 7 %; the more seldom causes like toxic drug damage, lesions in MS and paraneoplastic syndromes, vestibular migraine, vitamin B12 deficiency, or traumatic and hypoxic injuries occur in decreasing frequency (Wagner et al. 2008). It can, however, also be caused, but more seldom, by a paramedian lesion of the medulla oblongata, for example, in MS, hemorrhage, infarction, or tumor.

There are two subgroups of the idiopathic form of DBN:

• One appearing with clear cerebellar signs but without cerebellar pathology in MRI.
• The other in combination with bilateral vestibulopathy, peripheral polyneuropathy, or a cerebellar syndrome, suggesting a multisystem degeneration. In 89 % of patients with CANVAS (cerebellar ataxia with neuropathy and bilateral

vestibular areflexia syndrome), a circumscribed atrophy of the cerebellum of the anterior and dorsal vermis and crus I was seen in MRI (Kirchner et al. 2011; Szmulewicz et al. 2011; Wagner et al. 2008).

Upbeat Nystagmus (UBN)

Upbeat nystagmus (http://extra.springer.com) is rarer than DBN. It is a fixation-induced nystagmus that abruptly beats upward in primary gaze position and is par-tially dependent on head position. UBN is combined with a disorder of the vertical smooth pursuit eye movements, a visual and vestibulospinal ataxia with a tendency to fall backward, and past-pointing downward.

Pathoanatomical findings indicate that:

- Most acute lesions are located paramedially in the medulla oblongata, in neurons of the paramedian tract, close to the caudal part of the perihypoglossal nucleus, which is responsible for vertical gaze-holding (Janssen et al. 1998; Pierrot-Deseilligny et al. 2007).
- However, lesions have been reported to occur paramedially in the tegmentum of the pontomesencephalic junction, the brachium conjunctivum, and probably in the anterior vermis (Leigh and Zee 2006; Pierrot-Deseilligny et al. 2005).

There are also indications that a lateral lesion in the caudal pons, which includes the superior vestibular nucleus and its connection to the central ventral tegmental tract, CVTT, can lead to a UBN (Tiliket et al. 2008).

The symptoms persist as a rule for several weeks but are not permanent. Because the eye movements generally have larger amplitudes, oscillopsia in UBN is very distressing and impairs vision. UBN due to damage of the pontomesencephalic brainstem is frequently combined—especially in MS patients—with a unilateral or bilateral internuclear ophthalmoplegia (INO), indicating that the MLF is affected. The main etiologies are bilateral lesions in MS, brainstem ischemia or tumor (Fig. 3.8), Wernicke's encephalopathy, cerebellar degeneration, and dysfunction of the cerebellum due to intoxication.

Therapy for DBN and UBN

It is therapeutically expedient to try to treat the symptoms of persisting DBN with various drugs. In the last years the potassium channel blockers 3,4-diaminopyridine and 4-aminopyridine have been proven to have a positive effect, above all in DBN and also in single cases of UBN (Strupp et al. 2004; Kalla et al. 2004, 2007; Tsunemi et al. 2010) (Fig. 3.9). For this reason a therapeutic attempt can be made with $3 \times 5–10$ mg/day 4-aminopyridine (or $1–2 \times 10$ mg in the sustained release form) for DBN.

Animal experiments have shown that administration of aminopyridines can increase the resting-state activity and excitability of Purkinje cells (Etzion and Grossman 2001) and thus improve the reduced inhibitory GABA-mediated influence

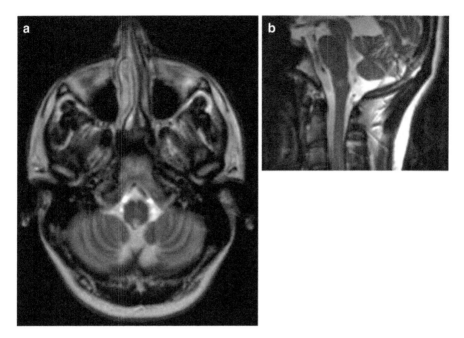

Fig. 3.8 Magnetic resonance tomography (with contrast medium) of a patient with upbeat nystagmus syndrome induced by a contrast-absorbing tumor located paramedially in the medulla oblongata (**a**) transversal slice and (**b**) sagittal slice

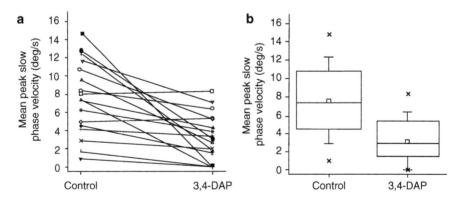

Fig. 3.9 Effect of 3,4-diaminopyridine on downbeat nystagmus: influence of 3,4-diaminopyridine (3,4-DAP) on the mean velocity of the slow phase of downbeat nystagmus (DBN, measured with 2-D video-oculography). The figures (**a**) through (**d**) show the mean velocity of the slow phase of DBN for each individual patient. (**a**) Controls versus 3,4-DAP and (**c**) controls versus placebo. Both graphs (**b**) and (**d**) show a so-called box plot with mean value, median, and 50 percentile as well as standard deviation for controls versus 3,4-DAP (**b**) and controls versus placebo (**d**). 3,4-DAP reduced the maximal velocity of the slow phase of DBN from 7.2°/s to 3.1°/s 30 min after ingestion of 20 mg 3, 4-DAP ($p < 0.001$). (**e**) shows an original recording of vertical eye position before and 30 min after ingestion of the medicine (reproduced with permission from Strupp et al. (2003))

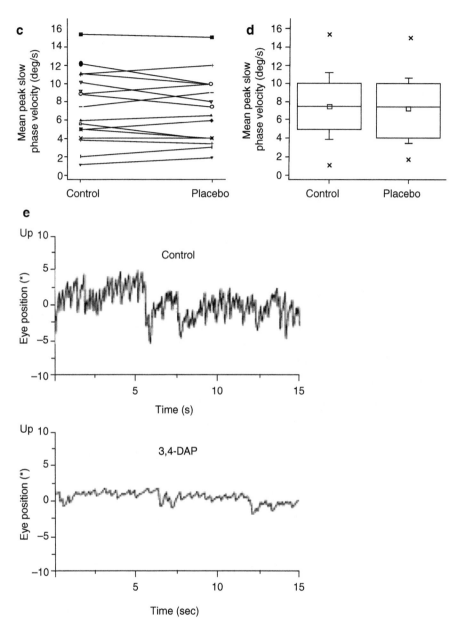

Fig. 3.9 (continued)

of the cerebellum on the superior vestibular nuclei. Since epileptic attacks or heart rhythm disorders—especially at higher dosages—can occur in rare cases, an ECG should be performed before and ca. 60 min after the first ingestion of 5 mg 4-aminopyridine in order to promptly detect any lengthening of the QT interval (Strupp et al. 2011a, b). This is so far a single, nonstandard therapeutic attempt.

Since generally UBN slowly resolves after an acute occurrence, therapy for its symptoms is often not necessary. In cases of very disturbing oscillopsias due to large amplitudes of the nystagmus or its longer duration, one can try 4-aminopyridine (3×5–10 mg/day orally) (Glasauer et al. 2005a) or memantine (2×10–20 mg/day) or gabapentin (3×300–600 mg/day orally) (Averbuch-Heller et al. 1997; Strack et al. 2010; Thurtell et al. 2010). If both are ineffective, one can try baclofen (2×5–10 mg/day orally) (Dieterich et al. 1991).

3.1.5.3 Central Vestibular Syndromes in the Vertical (Roll) Plane

- These syndromes indicate an acute unilateral injury of the "graviceptive" vestibular pathways in the brainstem: from the vertical canals and otoliths over the *ipsilateral* (medial and superior) vestibular nuclei and the *contralateral* MLF to the nuclei of the extraocular eye muscles and integration centers for vertical and torsional eye movements (INC and riMLF) in the rostral midbrain (Brandt and Dieterich 1994; Dieterich and Brandt 1992, 1993a, b, c). Unilateral lesions of the vestibulocerebellar structures (e.g., the uvula, nodulus, dentate nucleus) can also induce signs in the roll plane (Baier and Dieterich 2009).
- More rostral to the midbrain, only the vestibular projection of the VOR for perception in the roll plane (determination of the subjective visual vertical, SVV) runs over the vestibular nuclei in the posterolateral thalamus (Dieterich and Brandt 1993b) to the vestibular cortical network, especially the parietoinsular vestibular cortex (PIVC) in the posterior insula (Brandt and Dieterich 1994; Brandt et al. 1994) and the superior temporal gyrus (Baier et al. 2012b). Lesions rostral to the midbrain manifest with perceptual deficits only.
- Perceptual deficits in the sense of pathological deviations of the SVV occur during unilateral damage along the entire VOR projection and of the vestibulocerebellum. They are one of the most sensitive signs of acute brainstem or cerebellar lesions (in ca. 90 % of cases of acute unilateral infarctions) (Dieterich and Brandt 1993a; Baier et al. 2008; Baier and Dieterich 2009). Deviation of the SVV in the acute phase is more pronounced in patients with lesions in the region of the vestibular nuclei (Wallenberg's syndrome) than in patients with vestibular neuritis; this means an average of 9.8° as opposed to 7° (Cnyrim et al. 2007). The remission of the perceptual deficits over a period of ca. 2–4 weeks is very similar in both diseases (Fig. 3.5).
- The crossing of graviceptive pathways at pontine level is especially important for topographic diagnosis of brainstem disorders:
  All signs of lesions in the roll plane—single components or a complete ocular tilt reaction (http://extra.springer.com) (i.e., head tilt, vertical divergence of the eyes, ocular torsion, SVV deviation)—exhibit an *ipsiversive* tilt (ipsilateral eye lowermost) in cases of the very rare unilateral peripheral vestibular lesion and the frequent pontomedullary lesion (medial and superior vestibular nuclei) below the decussation in the brainstem.
  All signs in the roll plane—ocular motor, perceptual, and postural—exhibit *contraversive* deviations (contralateral eye lowermost) in cases of unilateral

pontomesencephalic lesions of the brainstem above the decussation and indicate damage to the MLF or of the supranuclear center of the INC.

- Lesions of the vestibular nucleus due to dorsolateral pontomedullary infarctions—Wallenberg's syndrome—represent a prototype of a vestibular tonus imbalance in the roll plane. It manifests with lateropulsion of the eyes and the body and single components or a complete ipsilateral ocular tilt reaction (Dieterich and Brandt 1993a, b, c).
- Brainstem lesions ipsilateral to the vestibular nucleus, near the ascending medial lemniscus (ipsilateral vestibulo-thalamic tract, IVTT), also induce isolated *ipsilateral* deviations of the SVV without vertical divergence or ocular torsion (Zwergal et al. 2008).
- Depending on the damaged region of the cerebellum, unilateral lesions of the vestibulocerebellum induce primarily contraversive (ca. 60 %) and more seldom (ca. 25 %) ipsiversive deviations (Baier et al. 2008; Baier and Dieterich 2009). The structure most frequently impaired in cases of contraversive signs is the dentate nucleus.
- Ocular tilt reaction in unilateral infarctions of the paramedian thalamus (in 50 %) is caused by a simultaneous lesion in the paramedian rostral midbrain (INC).
- Unilateral lesions of the paramedian and posterolateral thalamus can cause moderate ipsiversive or contraversive SVV tilt, which indicates damage to the so-called vestibular thalamic nuclei. Occasionally this tilt is combined with thalamic astasia and generally resolves within a matter of days or a few weeks.
- Acute unilateral lesions of the PIVC and of the superior temporal gyrus of the right or left hemisphere often lead to a vestibular function disorder with moderate ipsiversive, mostly contraversive SVV tilts lasting several days (Brandt et al. 1994; Barra et al. 2010; Baier et al. 2012b) (Fig. 3.10).
- Some of the patients with lesions of the PIVC, of the superior temporal gyrus, the operculum, and the anterior insula simultaneously show a pusher syndrome (Johannsen et al. 2006). There is a positive correlation between the extent of the pushing and the SVV deviation (Baier et al. 2012a). This occurs more frequently with lesions of the right hemisphere (42 %) than with lesions of the left hemisphere (25 %) and indicates a close connection between the control of posture and stance and the vestibular system (Fig. 3.11).
- If instead of a functional deficit due to a lesion, the VOR projection is stimulated on one side, the same effects will be triggered, but in the opposite direction.
- If a torsional nystagmus occurs in the acute phase, the rapid nystagmus phase will be in the opposite direction of the tonic skew deviation and the ocular torsion (Helmchen et al. 1998).

Complicated ocular motor syndromes are occasionally induced in midbrain lesions by the combination of:

- A central vestibular deficit in the roll plane (e.g., due to the INC deficit) and at the same time
- A nuclear or fascicular third nerve or fourth nerve palsy (Fig. 3.12)

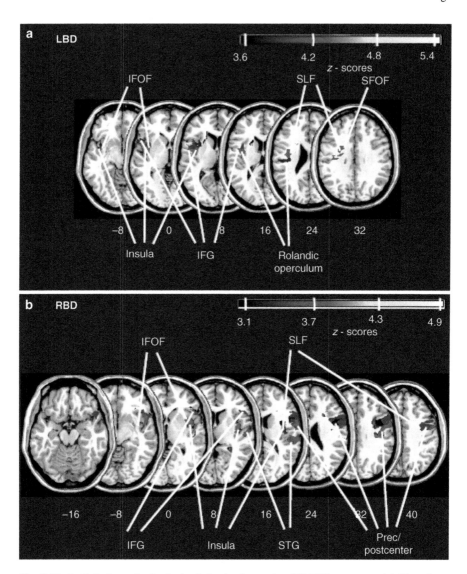

Fig. 3.10 Statistical voxel-wise lesion-behavioral mapping (VLBM) compares (**a**) 22 patients with a lesion of the left hemisphere with (**b**) 32 patients with a lesion of the right hemisphere as regards the absolute SVV deviations (*t*-test). Shown are all voxels that remain after correction for multiple comparisons with 1 % FDR (false discovery rate) threshold. SVV deviations are associated with lesions of the insula of both hemispheres as well as in addition with lesions in the superior temporal gyrus (*STG*) and the inferior frontal gyrus (*IFG*)

This leads to a "mixed pattern" that can nevertheless be clearly differentiated by determining the SVV, binocularly as well as for each individual eye separately (monocular measurement), and by measuring tonic ocular torsion by fundus photographs (Dichgans and Dieterich 1995). A central vestibular lesion induces in both eyes a contralateral SVV deviation of generally 10–20° in the same direction. If

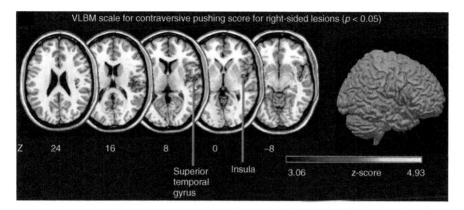

Fig. 3.11 Here is shown the statistical voxel-wise lesion-behavioral mapping (*VLBM*) used to compare the lesion site with the amount of pushing (scale for contraversive pushing in %) for right-brain lesions (FDR corrected alpha threshold $p < 0.05$). The lesion areas are located in the posterior insula, the superior temporal gyrus, and in the white matter

Fig. 3.12   Magnetic resonance image (T2-weighted, (**a**) coronal slices, (**b**) transversal slices) of a patient with a mixed pattern of ocular tilt reaction to the right and a lesion of the oculomotor nucleus and fascicle on the left due to an acute paramedian thalamus midbrain infarction, which was caused by a dissection of the left vertebral artery with embolism. The left-sided lesion encompasses in the upper midbrain the region of oculomotor nuclei with the fascicle as well as the supranuclear ocular motor and vestibular centers of the interstitial nucleus of Cajal (INC) and the rostral interstitial nucleus of the medial longitudinal fascicle (riMLF). One month after the infarction, the deviation of the subjective visual vertical (SVV) still amounted to +4–5° for the ipsilateral left eye and +8–10° for the contralateral right eye; fundus photography showed an incyclorotation of the left eye of 4° and an excyclorotation of the right eye of 7°. There was additional gaze palsy for upward and downward directions

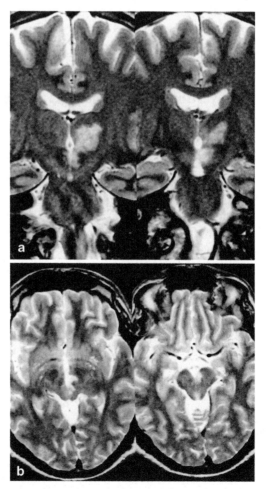

there is also an oculomotor or trochlear lesion—mostly in one eye—the SVV deviation in the affected eye will be reduced or even antagonized, with the result that the SVV deviation clearly differs for both eyes or even points in totally opposite directions and the affected eye in addition looks in the ipsilateral direction (mixed pattern).

By measuring the SVV for each eye separately (monocular), the peripheral infranuclear oculomotor and trochlear palsies, which appear to be clinically similar, can also be differentiated from central vestibular syndromes, as infranuclear palsies cannot induce any SVV deviation or ocular torsion in both eyes (Dieterich and Brandt 1993c). Even the Bielschowsky head-tilt test does not allow clear differentiation between a trochlear palsy (http://extra.springer.com) and an ocular tilt reaction.

The etiology of these unilateral lesions is frequently an infarction as well as hemorrhage of the brainstem or of the paramedian thalamus, which extends into the rostral midbrain (Dieterich and Brandt 1993a, b). The course and prognosis depend also here on the etiology of the underlying illness. In the frequent ischemias, one can expect a significant and most often complete recovery from the symptoms in the roll plane within days to weeks due to central compensation taking place over the opposite unaffected side (Dieterich and Brandt 1992, 1993b; Cnyrim et al. 2007) (Fig. 3.5).

3.2   Vestibular Migraine/Migraine of the Basilar Type

3.2.1   Patient History

The main symptoms of migraine as a subform of migraine of the basilar type are:

- Recurring attacks of various combinations of vertigo and ataxia of stance and gait
- Visual disorders and other brainstem symptoms, accompanied or followed by occipital head pressure or headache
- Nausea and vomiting.

Aura symptoms last for 5–60 min (ICHD 2004). As any movement increases the complaints, patients often have a need for rest. The attacks can, however, take a monosymptomatic course, manifesting with only vertigo and perhaps also with a hearing disorder in the sense of a vestibular migraine. The monosymptomatic, audiovestibular attacks with the main symptom of vertigo predominate in ca. 75 % of such cases and are called vestibular migraine (Dieterich and Brandt 1999; Strupp et al. 2010).

3.2.2 Clinical Aspects and Course

If vertigo was the key symptom of the migraine, it was also alternatively called "migrainous vertigo" (Neuhauser et al. 2001; Neuhauser and Lempert 2004) or "migraine-associated vertigo" (Brantberg et al. 2005) or migraine-related vestibulopathy. Over the last years the term "vestibular migraine" has prevailed, increasingly becoming established in the international literature (Radtke et al. 2011). In the meantime the diagnostic criteria of *vestibular migraine* have been defined in a consensus document of the International Headache Society and the Bárány Society (Lempert et al. 2012).

The diagnosis is simple if the attacks are generally or always followed by headache (or occipital head pressure) and if there is a positive family or personal history of other types of migraine (ca. 50 %; Dieterich and Brandt 1999). The occurrence of symptoms like light and sound hypersensitivity, need for quiet, tiredness after the attack, and urge to urinate also makes diagnosis easier. The attacks are more difficult to recognize if headache is absent (in ca. 30 %; Dieterich and Brandt 1999). The duration of the attacks of vertigo varies greatly and lasts either only seconds to minutes or several hours to days (Cutrer and Baloh 1992; Dieterich and Brandt 1999; Neuhauser et al. 2001; Radtke et al. 2012). Stress, hormone fluctuations, and sleep deficiency can trigger attacks as in migraine without aura (Lempert et al. 2009). Helpful for the diagnosis is the fact that contrary to other forms of migraine, 45–63 % of persons with vestibular migraine also show slight central ocular motor disorders in the form of:

- Gaze-evoked nystagmus (sometimes dissociated)
- A saccadic smooth pursuit beyond age norm (especially vertical)
- A spontaneous horizontal or vertical nystagmus
- A central positional nystagmus (Dieterich and Brandt 1999; Radtke et al. 2012; Neugebauer et al. 2013).

A pathological nystagmus is frequently observed during an attack, e.g., a central positional nystagmus, which in ca. 50 % of the cases can be attributed to a central vestibular dysfunction and in 15 %, to a peripheral vestibular dysfunction (von Brevern et al. 2005). The patients are generally hypersensitive to movement and motion sickness, particularly during the migraine attack (Cutrer and Baloh 1992). Like phonophobia and photophobia during migraine attacks, this hypersensitivity to movement is possibly induced by a sensory neuron overexcitability, here, for example, of the inner-ear receptors. Such overexcitability has been included in the diagnostic criteria (Neuhauser et al. 2001; Lempert et al. 2012).

The symptoms in most monosymptomatic audiovestibular cases with isolated vertigo do not fulfill the criteria of the International Headache Society (IHS) for a migraine of basilar type; it requires at least two aura symptoms of the posterior vascular territories, which normally develop within 5–20 min and last no longer than 60 min (IHS 2004). Frequently, however, the attacks of vestibular migraine are shorter or longer, or the attack is only monosymptomatic. For these reasons, the diagnostic criteria for vestibular migraine proposed by Neuhauser and coworkers (2001) have been agreed upon. They are based on the combination of attacks of vertigo and associated migraine symptoms. The novel diagnostic criteria of the consensus document (Lempert et al. 2012) are based on these (Overview 3.2).

Overview 3.2 Diagnostic Criteria for Vestibular Migraine (Consensus Document of the Bárány Society and the International Headache Society; Lempert et al. 2012)

1. *Vestibular Migraine*

   A. At least five episodes with vestibular symptoms of moderate or severe intensity, lasting 5 min to 72 h
   B. Current or previous history of migraine with or without aura according to the International Classification of Headache Disorders (ICHD 2004)
   C. One or more migraine features with at least 50 % of vestibular episodes:

      • Headache with at least two of the following characteristics: one-sided location, pulsating quality, moderate or severe pain intensity, and aggravation by routine physical activity
      • Photophobia and phonophobia
      • Visual aura

   D. Not better accounted for by another vestibular or ICHD diagnosis

2. *Probable Vestibular Migraine*

   A. At least five episodes with vestibular symptoms of moderate or severe intensity, lasting 5 min to 72 h
   B. Only one of the criteria B and C for vestibular migraine is fulfilled (migraine history *or* migraine features during the episode)
   C. Not better accounted for by another vestibular or ICHD diagnosis

A long-term evaluation of the criteria for a definitive or a possible migraine (Neuhauser et al. 2001) was conducted in a recent study involving 75 patients (Radtke et al. 2011, 2012). The follow-up examination took place in the eighth year (8.75 ± 1.3 years) since the diagnosis was established. Half of the patients diagnosed to have possible vestibular migraine developed a definitive vestibular migraine in the course of the illness. In 85 % of the patients with a diagnosis of definitive vestibular migraine, the diagnosis was confirmed, i.e., the diagnosis could be established with a high validity on the basis of the clinical criteria. Eight patients had developed a slight bilateral sensorineural hearing disorder that could have formally fulfilled the criteria for a bilateral Menière's disease, but they did not have the typical attacks. In individual cases this makes it difficult to separate the two diseases and in clinical practice leads to treatment of both (e.g., migraine prophylaxis plus betahistine). The frequency of central ocular motor signs over time increased from 15 to 41 % (Radtke et al. 2012).

Originally, Bickerstaff described migraine of the basilar type in 1961 as a typical illness of adolescence, which clearly predominates in females. Retrospective studies have, however, shown that migraine of the basilar type with dizziness and vestibular migraine can develop throughout a patient's entire life, most often in young adults but also between the sixth and seventh decades (Dieterich and Brandt 1999; Neuhauser et al. 2001; Lempert and Neuhauser 2009; Strupp et al. 2010). The ratio of women to men affected is 1.5:1.

Both vertigo and migraine without aura frequently occur in the population. The lifetime prevalence of vertigo is 7 % and that of migraine, up to 16 %. A coincidental, simultaneous occurrence of the two can be expected in 1.1 %; however, newer epidemiological examinations have shown this actually occurs in 3.2 % of the general population (Lempert and Neuhauser 2009). In part this co-occurrence can be explained by the fact that patients with migraine frequently have various vertigo syndromes, e.g., BPPV, Menière's disease (Radtke et al. 2002), or somatoform phobic postural vertigo (Best et al. 2009). The frequency of an actual vestibular migraine in dedicated dizziness outpatient clinics is about 10 % (Dieterich and Brandt 1999; Neuhauser et al. 2001; Strupp et al. 2010) and at least 9 % in headache outpatient clinics (Lempert and Neuhauser 2009). The lifetime prevalence of vestibular migraine is around 1 %, and the 1-year prevalence is 0.89 % (Neuhauser et al. 2006). Migraine without aura naturally has a higher 1-year prevalence of 12–14 % after puberty in women, whereas it is 7–8 % in men. Women are affected two to three times more often than men.

If the attacks in childhood take a monosymptomatic course without headache, they cannot be differentiated clinically from benign paroxysmal vertigo in childhood. The latter is considered to be equivalent to migraine with attacks that begin between the first and fourth year of life, last only seconds to minutes, and disappear spontaneously within a few years.

3.2.3 Pathophysiology and Therapeutic Principles

As to the pathogenesis of vestibular migraine, it is interesting that the rare episodic ataxia type 2 (due to a mutation of the PQ calcium channel gene on chromosome 19p13) occurs together with hemiplegic migraine in several families. The gene for hemiplegic migraine is also located on chromosome 19p13 (Ophoff et al. 1996). In the meantime three causative genes are known to induce the familial forms of hemiplegic migraine (FHM): FHM1, CACNA1A; FHM2, ATP1A2; and FHM3, SCN1A (De Fusco et al. 2003; Dichgans et al. 2005). Moreover, central ocular motor findings during the symptom-free interval in patients with vestibular migraine, as in episodic ataxia, also point to hereditary neuronal function disorders in the brainstem nuclei (channelopathies?). Neuronal functional disorders in the brainstem are also being discussed as factors in the pathophysiology of migraine without

aura. Animal studies have identified the locus coeruleus in the pontine brainstem—
the most important central core of the noradrenergic system—to be the modulator
of the cerebral blood flow in this primarily neurovascular headache syndrome, in
which the trigeminovascular system along with neurogenic inflammatory reactions
plays a central role (Goadsby 2000). Furthermore, the serotonergic dorsal raphe
nucleus in the midbrain seems to play an important role. Positron emission tomography studies have shown that this region and that of the dorsal pons with the locus
coeruleus are also activated in patients during migraine attacks without aura (Weiller
et al. 1995). These brainstem nuclei are also activated immediately after successful
treatment of a migraine attack, but not during the symptom-free interval. Drug therapy for migraine without aura acts at various sites within the trigeminovascular
system and the neurogenic inflammatory cascade.

Another pathogenetic approach has to do with cortical "spreading depression" as
a cause of aura. Here the vestibular symptoms could be eventually classified as
brainstem aura in the sense of a non-cortical spreading depression (Furman et al.
2003). This fits findings of an animal study that was able to prove a spreading
depression in the brainstem of rats on the basis of changes in the local brain circulation as well as systemic blood pressure (Richter et al. 2008). Likewise a migraine-
induced ischemia in the brainstem and labyrinth could be attributed to vasospasm.
The transient relapsing ischemia in the labyrinth could, on the other hand, explain
an endolymphatic hydrops and consequently Menière-similar symptoms as well
as BPPV, both of which frequently occur in association with vestibular migraine
(Lee et al. 2000; Radtke et al. 2002).

3.2.4 Pragmatic Therapy

So far the results of prospective, controlled studies are not available. Therapy analogous to that for migraine without aura was introduced, and the same principles have
proven valid both for treatment of the attacks of migraine and for their prophylaxis.
The symptoms of dizziness and the accompanying headache can, however, react
differently to the therapy or prophylaxis.

3.2.4.1 Stopping Attacks

To stop attacks lasting 45 min and longer, it is advisable to administer early
an antiemetic (e.g., metoclopramide, domperidone) in combination with a
nonsteroidal anti-inflammatory agent (e.g., ibuprofen, diclofenac) or an analgesic
(acetylsalicylic acid as a soluble tablet or paracetamol as a suppository).

In individual cases the triptans had positive effects on attacks of vertigo, acting
at the $5-HT_{1B/1D}$ receptors of the arteries (Bikhazi et al. 1997). Zolmitriptan, however, which was investigated in a randomized, placebo-controlled study, did not
have a positive effect in patients with vestibular migraine (Neuhauser et al. 2003).

3.2.4.2 Migraine Prophylaxis

The treatment of first choice for migraine prophylaxis is the administration of the beta-receptor blocker metoprolol retard (ca. 100 mg/day, e.g., in the evening) for about 6 months. Alternatives are topiramate (50–150 mg/day) and valproic acid (600–1,200 mg/day). However, good prospective, randomized studies have not yet been performed on any of these drugs. Mostly only observations have been made in a small number of cases. In a retrospective study in 100 patients with vestibular migraine, it was found that the 74 who received one of the above-mentioned drugs as migraine prophylaxis experienced a significant improvement of the duration, intensity, and frequency of their vertigo attacks as well as the associated migraine symptoms (Baier et al. 2009a).

3.2.4.3 Ineffective Treatments

The sole use of opioids, antivertiginous drugs (dimenhydrinate), or some anticonvulsants such as carbamazepine, diphenylhydantoin, and primidone is ineffective for vestibular migraine attacks.

3.2.5 Differential Diagnosis and Clinical Problems

Occasionally it can be difficult to differentiate vestibular migraine from:

- Transient ischemic attacks
- Menière's disease
- Vestibular paroxysmia
- Episodic ataxia type 2.

In some cases the diagnosis can only be established on the basis of the response to a "specific" therapy. Transitional and mixed forms or pathophysiological combinations are currently being discussed (see above), especially for Menière's disease and vestibular migraine. This would fit with findings that a higher percentage of patients with vestibular migraine as well as those with Menière's disease (68–70 %) mostly have bilateral damage to the labyrinth in the form of a significant reduction of the amplitude of sacculus-mediated cervical vestibular-evoked myogenic potentials (Baier et al. 2009b). Currently there are no reliable data, in part because patients with primarily vestibular symptoms are probably more frequently misdiagnosed as having Menière's disease. This would explain the considerable difference in prevalence of migraine in patients with "classic" Menière's disease (22 %) as opposed to "vestibular" Menière's disease (81 %) (Rassekh and Harker 1992). An interview-based study involving 78 patients with confirmed unilateral or bilateral Menière's disease determined that the lifetime prevalence of migraine with and without aura is 56 % compared with 25 % in an age-matched control group (Radtke et al. 2002). These figures suggest that there is either a pathophysiological link between the two diseases or alternatively the current diagnostic criteria cannot yet differentiate between them, or both are possible.

As BPPV occurs three times more frequently in migraine patients than in trauma patients according to a retrospective study (Ishiyama et al. 2000), it has been speculated that a relapsing functional deficit of the inner ear may be the underlying cause of the vestibular migraine attacks (e.g., in the form of a vasospasm). The therapy for BPPV in migraine patients is similar to the liberatory maneuvers used to treat idiopathic BPPV.

Episodic ataxia type 2 (see also Sect. 6.1.4) is also characterized by episodic attacks of dizziness with central ocular motor deficits especially downbeat nystagmus, even during the attack-free interval (Griggs and Nutt 1995). It is an autosomal dominant disorder caused by mutation in the calcium channel gene CACNA1A (Ophoff et al. 1996), mainly impairing the function of cerebellar Purkinje cells. The reduced calcium current of the inhibitory Purkinje cells causes a disinhibition of cerebellar nuclei resulting in these attacks of ataxia and ocular motor disturbances. A placebo-controlled study showed that administration of 4-aminopyridine is effective (Strupp et al. 2011a, b). Empirical use of acetazolamide has also proven successful.

An early differential diagnosis is particularly important for vestibular migraine patients because:

- They develop a somatoform vertigo significantly more often than patients with other vestibular syndromes.
- Comorbidities of up to 65 % occur with somatoform disorders (like pathological anxiety and depression) (Eckhardt-Henn et al. 2008).
- The patients often feel themselves more impaired in their daily life.
- They especially perceive their vestibular symptoms much stronger and have more anxiety (Best et al. 2009).

Patients with somatoform vertigo (see also Chap. 5) describe postural or diffuse dizziness (light-headedness, feeling of emptiness in the head, etc.) more often, while at the same time, they have normal findings in the neuro-otological tests. Depending on the underlying psychiatric disorder, additional symptoms will be present:

- Motivation and concentration disorders
- Decline of performance
- Subjectively experienced restrictions in professional and everyday activities
- Vegetative symptoms that accompany the vertigo symptoms (tachycardia, nausea, profuse sweating, dyspnea, fear of suffocating, loss of appetite, weight loss)
- Disorders of mood
- Sleep disorders
- Symptoms of anxiety.

Important differential diagnoses that must be quickly clarified are:

- Transient ischemic attacks in the vertebrobasilar system
- Basilar artery thrombosis

- Brainstem/cerebellum hemorrhage, which can also accompany headache centered primarily in the nuchal region.

Basilar artery thrombosis and brainstem hemorrhage usually develop quite rapidly, along with:

- Vigilance disorders that can worsen until coma
- Increasing deficits of the cranial nerves
- Paresis or sensory deficits in the extremities.

A vertebral artery dissection can occur spontaneously or after head trauma or chiropractic maneuvers. It is associated with occipital head and nuchal pain, nuchal pressure, dizziness, and other brainstem symptoms. As smaller brainstem ischemias can be induced in the context of various mechanisms, it is especially important to consider the possibility of the more dangerous life-threatening brainstem ischemia in the differential diagnosis at the appearance of the first migraine attack or first three migraine attacks.

References

Anagnostou E, Spengos K, Vassilopoulou S, Paraskevas GP, Zis V, Vassilopoulos D. Incidence of rotational vertigo in supratentorial stroke: a prospective analysis of 112 consecutive patients. J Neurol Sci. 2010;290:33–6.

Averbuch-Heller L, Tusa RJ, Fuhry L, Rottach KG, Ganser GL, Heide W, et al. A double-blind controlled study of gabapentin and baclofen as treatment for acquired nystagmus. Ann Neurol. 1997;41:818–25.

Baier B, Dieterich M. Ocular tilt reaction – a clinical sign of cerebellar infarctions? Neurology. 2009;72:572–3.

Baier B, Bense S, Dieterich M. Are signs of ocular tilt reaction in patients with cerebellar lesions mediated by the dentate nucleus? Brain. 2008;131:1445–54.

Baier B, Winkenwerder E, Dieterich M. Vestibular migraine: effects of prophylactic therapy. J Neurol. 2009a;256(3):426–32.

Baier B, Stieber N, Dieterich M. Vestibular-evoked myogenic potentials in "vestibular migraine". J Neurol. 2009b;256(9):1447–54.

Baier B, Janzen J, Fechir M, Müller N, Dieterich M. Pusher syndrome – its anatomical correlate. J Neurol. 2012a;259:277–83.

Baier B, Suchan J, Karnath HO, Dieterich M. Neuronal correlate of verticality perception – a voxelwise lesion study. Neurology. 2012b;78(10):728–35.

Barra J, Marquer A, Joassin R, Reymond C, Metge L, Chauvineau V, et al. Humans use internal models to construct and update sense of verticality. Brain. 2010;133:3552–63.

Bense S, Best C, Buchholz HG, Wiener V, Schreckenberger M, Bartenstein P, et al. 18F-fluorodeoxyglucose hypometabolism in cerebellar tonsil and flocculus in downbeat-nystagmus. Neuroreport. 2006;17:599–603.

Best C, Eckhardt-Henn A, Tschan R, Bense S, Dieterich M. Psychiatric morbidity and comorbidity in different vestibular vertigo syndromes: results of a prospective longitudinal study over one year. J Neurol. 2009;256:58–65.

Bickerstaff ER. Basilar artery migraine. Lancet. 1961;I:15–7.

Bikhazi P, Jackson C, Ruckenstein MJ. Efficacy of antimigrainous therapy in the treatment of migraine-associated dizziness. Am J Otol. 1997;18:350.

Brandt T. Cortical matching of visual and vestibular 3-D coordinate maps. Ann Neurol. 1997; 42:983–4.

Brandt T. Vertigo: its multisensory syndromes. 2nd ed. London: Springer; 1999.

Brandt T, Dieterich M. Vestibular syndromes in the roll plane: topographic diagnosis from brainstem to cortex. Ann Neurol. 1994;36:337–47.

Brandt T, Dieterich M. Central vestibular syndromes in roll, pitch, and yaw planes. Topographic diagnosis of brainstem disorders. Neuroophthalmology. 1995;15:291–303.

Brandt T, Dieterich M. The vestibular cortex: its locations, functions, and disorders. Ann N Y Acad Sci. 1999;871:293–312.

Brandt T, Dieterich M, Büchele W. Postural abnormalities in central vestibular brain stem lesions. In: Bles W, Brandt T, editors. Disorders of posture and gait. Amsterdam/New York/Oxford: Elsevier; 1986. p. 141–56.

Brandt T, Dieterich M, Danek A. Vestibular cortex lesions affect the perception of verticality. Ann Neurol. 1994;35:528–34.

Brandt T, Bötzel K, Yousry T, Dieterich M, Schulze S. Rotational vertigo in embolic stroke of the vestibular and auditory cortices. Neurology. 1995;45:42–4.

Brandt T, Dieterich M, Strupp M, Glasauer S. Model approach to neurological variants of visuo-spatial neglect. Biol Cybern. 2012;106:681–90.

Brantberg K, Trees N, Baloh RW. Migraine-associated vertigo. Acta Otolaryngol. 2005; 125:276–9.

Büttner U, Helmchen C, Büttner-Ennever JA. The localizing value of nystagmus in brainstem disorders. Neuroophthalmology. 1995;15:283–90.

Büttner-Ennever JA. Mapping the oculomotor system. Prog Brain Res. 2008;171:3–11.

Chen A, DeAngelis GC, Angelaki DE. Convergence of vestibular and visual self-motion signals in an area of the posterior sylvian fissure. J Neurosci. 2011;31:11617–27.

Cnyrim CD, Rettinger N, Mansmann U, Brandt T, Strupp M. Central compensation of deviated subjective visual vertical in Wallenberg's syndrome. J Neurol Neurosurg Psychiatry. 2007;78:527–8.

Cnyrim CD, Newman-Toker D, Karch C, Brandt T, Strupp M. Beside differentiation of vestibular neuritis from central "vestibular pseudoneuritis". J Neurol Neurosurg Psychiatry. 2008;79:458–60.

Cutrer FM, Baloh RW. Migraine-associated dizziness. Headache. 1992;32:300–4.

De Fusco M, Marconi R, Silvestri L, et al. Haploinsufficiency of ATP1A2 encoding the Na+/K+ pump alpha2 subunit associated with familial hemiplegic migraine type 2. Nat Genet. 2003; 33:92–196.

Dichgans M, Dieterich M. Third nerve palsy with contralateral ocular torsion and binocular tilt of visual vertical, indicating a midbrain lesion. Neuroophthalmology. 1995;15:315–20.

Dichgans M, Freilinger T, Eckstein G, Babini E, Lorenz-Depiereux B, Biskup S, et al. Mutation in the neuronal voltage-gated sodium channel SCN1A in familial hemiplegic migraine. Lancet. 2005;366:371–7.

Dieterich M, Brandt T. Wallenberg's syndrome: lateropulsion, cyclorotation, and subjective visual vertical in thirty-six patients. Ann Neurol. 1992;31:399–408.

Dieterich M, Brandt T. Ocular torsion and tilt of subjective visual vertical are sensitive brainstem signs. Ann Neurol. 1993a;33:292–9.

Dieterich M, Brandt T. Thalamic infarctions: differential effects on vestibular function in roll plane (35 patients). Neurology. 1993b;43:1732–40.

Dieterich M, Brandt T. Ocular torsion and perceived vertical in oculomotor, trochlear and abducens nerve palsies. Brain. 1993c;116:1095–104.

Dieterich M, Brandt T. Episodic vertigo related to migraine (90 cases): vestibular migraine? J Neurol. 1999;246:883–92.

Dieterich M, Brandt T. Functional brain imaging of peripheral and central vestibular disorders. Brain. 2008;131:2538–52.

Dieterich M, Straube A, Brandt T, Paulus W, Büttner U. The effects of baclofen and cholinergic drugs on upbeat and downbeat nystagmus. J Neurol Neurosurg Psychiatry. 1991; 54:627–32.

Dieterich M, Grünbauer M, Brandt T. Direction-specific impairment of motion perception and spatial orientation in downbeat and upbeat nystagmus in humans. Neurosci Lett. 1998; 245:29–32.

Dieterich M, Bense S, Lutz S, Drzega A, Stephan T, Bartenstein P, et al. Dominance for vestibular cortical function in the non-dominant hemisphere. Cereb Cortex. 2003;13:994–1007.

Eckhardt-Henn A, Best C, Bense S, Breuer P, Diener G, Tschan R, et al. Psychiatric comorbidity in different organic vertigo syndromes. J Neurol. 2008;255:420–8.

Etzion Y, Grossman Y. Highly 4-aminopyridine sensitive delayed rectifier current modulates the excitability of guinea pig cerebellar Purkinje cells. Exp Brain Res. 2001;139:419–25.

Furman JM, Marcus DA, Balaban CD. Migrainous vertigo: development of a pathogenetic model and structured diagnostic interview. Curr Opin Neurol. 2003;16:5–13.

Glasauer S, Hoshi M, Kempermann U, Eggert T, Büttner U. Three-dimensional eye position and slow phase velocity in humans with downbeat nystagmus. J Neurophysiol. 2003;89:338–54.

Glasauer S, Kalla R, Büttner U, Strupp M, Brandt T. 4-aminopyridine restores visual ocular motor function in upbeat nystagmus. J Neurol Neurosurg Psychiatry. 2005a;76:451–3.

Glasauer S, Strupp M, Kalla R, Büttner U, Brandt T. Effect of 4-aminopyridine on upbeat and downbeat nystagmus elucidates the mechanism of downbeat nystagmus. Ann NY Acad Sci. 2005b;1039:528–31.

Goadsby PJ. The pharmacology of headache. Prog Neurobiol. 2000;62:509–25.

Goodale MA. Transforming vision into action. Vision Res. 2011;51:1567–87.

Griggs RC, Nutt JG. Episodic ataxias as channelopathies. Ann Neurol. 1995;37:285–7.

Grüsser OJ, Pause M, Schreiter U. Localization and responses of neurons in the parieto-insular vestibular cortex of the awake monkeys (Macaca fascicularis). J Physiol. 1990a;430: 537–57.

Grüsser OJ, Pause M, Schreiter U. Vestibular neurons in the parieto-insular vestibular cortex of monkeys (Macaca fascicularis): visual and neck receptor responses. J Physiol. 1990b;430: 559–83.

Halmagyi GM, Leigh RJ. Upbeat about downbeat nystagmus. Neurology. 2004;63:606–7.

Helmchen C, Rambold H, Fuhry L, Büttner U. Deficits in vertical and torsional eye movements after uni- and bilateral muscimol inactivation of the interstitial nucleus of Cajal of the alert monkey. Exp Brain Res. 1998;119:436–52.

Hewett R, Guye M, Gavaret M, Bartolomei F. Benign temporo-parieto-occipital junction epilepsy with vestibular disturbances: an underrecognized form of epilepsy? Epilepsy Behav. 2011; 21:412–6.

Hopf HC. Vertigo and masseter paresis. A new local brain-stem syndrome probably of vascular origin. J Neurol. 1987;235:42–5.

Hüfner K, Stephan T, Kalla R, Deutschländer A, Wagner J, Holtmannspötter M, et al. Structural and functional MRIs disclose cerebellar pathologies in idiopathic downbeat nystagmus. Neurology. 2007;69:1128–35.

International Headache Society Classification Subcommittee. International classification of headache disorders, 2nd edition. Cephalalgia. 2004;24:1–160.

Ishiyama A, Jacobson KM, Baloh RW. Migraine and benign positional vertigo. Otol Rhinol Laryngol. 2000;109:377–80.

Janssen JC, Larner AJ, Morris H, Bronstein AM, Farmer SF. Upbeat nystagmus: clinicoanatomical correlation. J Neurol Neurosurg Psychiatry. 1998;65:380–1.

Johannsen L, Fruhmann Berger M, Karnath HO. Subjective visual vertical (SVV) determined in a representative sample of 15 patients with pusher syndrome. J Neurol. 2006;253: 1367–9.

Kalla R, Glasauer S, Schautzer F, Lehnen N, Büttner U, Strupp M, et al. 4-Aminopyridine improved downbeat-nystagmus, smooth pursuit, and VOR-gain. Neurology. 2004;62: 1228–9.

Kalla R, Deutschländer A, Hüfner K, Stephan T, Jahn K, Glasauer S, et al. Detection of floccular hypometabolism in downbeat nystagmus by fMRI. Neurology. 2006;66:281–3.

Kalla R, Glasauer S, Büttner U, Brandt T, Strupp M. 4-Aminopyridine restores vertical and horizontal neural integrator function in downbeat nystagmus. Brain. 2007;130:2441–50.

Karnath HO, Rorden C. The anatomy of spatial neglect. Neuropsychologia. 2012;50:1010–7.

Kattah JC, Talkad AV, Wang DZ, et al. HINTS to diagnose stroke in acute vestibular syndrome. Three-step bedside oculomotor examination more sensitive than early MRI diffusion-weighted imaging. Stroke. 2009;40:3504–10.

Kim HA, Lee H. Isolated vestibular nucleus infarction mimicking acute peripheral vestibulopathy. Stroke. 2010;41:558–60.

Kirchner H, Kremmyda O, Hüfner K, Stephan T, Zingler V, Brandt T, et al. Clinical, electrophysiological, and MRI findings in patients with cerebellar ataxia and a bilaterally pathological head-impulse test. Ann NY Acad Sci. 2011;1233:127–38.

Lee H, Lopez I, Ishiyama A, Baloh RW. Can migraine damage the inner ear? Arch Neurol. 2000;57:1631–4.

Lee CC, Suy C, Ho HC, Hung SK, Lee MS, Chou P, et al. Risk of stroke in patients hospitalized for isolated vertigo. A four year follow-up study. Stroke. 2011;42:48–52.

Leigh RJ, Zee DS. The neurology of eye movements. 4th ed. New York/Oxford: Oxford University Press; 2006.

Lempert T, Neuhauser H. Epidemiology of vertigo, migraine and vestibular migraine. J Neurol. 2009;256(3):333–8.

Lempert T, Neuhauser H, Daroff RB. Vertigo as a symptom of migraine. Ann NY Acad Sci. 2009;1164:242–51.

Lempert T, Olesen J, Furman J, Waterston J, Seemungal B, Carey J, et al. Vestibular migraine: diagnostic criteria. Consensus document of the Barany Society and the International Headache Society. J Vest Res. 2012;22:167–72.

Marti S, Straumann D, Glasauer S. The origin of downbeat-nystagmus: an asymmetry in the distribution of on-directions of vertical gaze-velocity Purkinje-cells. Ann NY Acad Sci. 2005;1039:548–53.

Milner AD, Goodale MA. The visual brain in action. Oxford: Oxford University Press; 1995.

Naganuma M, Inatomi Y, Yonehara F, Fujioka S, Hashimoto Y, Hirano T, et al. Rotational vertigo associated with parietal cortical infarction. J Neurol Sci. 2006;246:159–61.

Neugebauer H, Adrion C, Glaser M, Strupp M. Long-term changes of central ocular motor signs in patients with vestibular migraine. Eur Neurol. 2013;69:102–7.

Neuhauser H, Lempert T. Vertigo and dizziness related to migraine: a diagnostic challenge. Cephalalgia. 2004;24:83–91.

Neuhauser H, Leopold M, von Brevern M, Arnold G, Lempert T. The interrelations of migraine, vertigo and migrainous vertigo. Neurology. 2001;56:436–41.

Neuhauser H, Radtke A, von Brevern M, Lempert T. Zolmitriptan for treatment of migrainous vertigo: a pilot randomised placebo-controlled trial. Neurology. 2003;60:882–3.

Neuhauser H, Radtke A, von Brevern M, Feldmann M, Lezius F, Ziese T, et al. Migrainous vertigo: prevalence and impact on quality of life. Neurology. 2006;67:1028–33.

Newman-Toker DE, Kattah JC, Alvernia JE, Wang DZ. Normal head impulse test differentiates acute cerebellar strokes from vestibular neuritis. Neurology. 2008;70:2378–85.

Ophoff RA, Terwindt GM, Vergouwe MN, van Eijk R, Oefner PJ, Hoffman SM, et al. Familial hemiplegic migraine and episodic ataxia type-2 are caused by mutations in the Ca2+ channel gene CACNA1A4. Cell. 1996;87:543–52.

Pierrot-Deseilligny C, Milea D. Vertical nystagmus: clinical facts and hypotheses. Brain. 2005; 128:1237–46.

Pierrot-Deseilligny C, Milea D, Sirmai J, Papeix C, Rivaud-Pechoux S. Upbeat nystagmus due to a small pontine lesion: evidence for the existence of a crossing ventral tegmental tract. Eur Neurol. 2005;54:186–90.

Pierrot-Deseilligny C, Richeh W, Bolgert F. Upbeat nystagmus due to a caudal medullary lesion influenced by gravity. J Neurol. 2007;254:120–1.

Radtke A, Lempert T, Gresty MA, Brookes GB, Bronstein AM, Neuhauser H. Migraine and Meniere's disease. Is there a link? Neurology. 2002;59:1700–4.

Radtke A, Neuhauser H, von Brevern M, et al. Vestibular migraine – validity of clinical diagnostic criteria. Cephalalgia 2011;31:906–13.

Radtke A, von Brevern M, Neuhauser H, Hottenrott T, Lempert T. Vestibular migraine. Long-term follow-up of clinical symptoms and vestibulo-cochlear findings. Neurology. 2012;79: 1607–14.

Rassekh CH, Harker LA. The prevalence of migraine in Meniere's disease. Laryngoscope. 1992;102:135–8.

Richter F, Bauer R, Lehmenkühler A, Schaible HG. Spreading depression in the brainstem of the adult rat: electrophysiological parameters and influences on regional brainstem blood flow. J Cereb Blood Flow Metab. 2008;28:984–94.

Sander T, Sprenger A, Mart S, Naumann T, Straumann D, Helmchen C. Effect of 4-aminopyridine on gravity dependence and neural integrator function in patients with idiopathic downbeat nystagmus. J Neurol. 2011;258:618–22.

Sierra-Hidalgo F, Pablo-Fernandez E, Herrero-San Martin A, Correas-Callero E, Herreros-Rodriguez J, Romero-Munoz JP, et al. Clinical and imaging features of the room tilt illusion. J Neurol. 2012;259(12):2555–64.

Spiegel R, Rettinger N, Kalla R, Lehnen N, Straumann D, Glasauer S, et al. The intensity of downbeat nystagmus during daytime. Ann NY Acad Sci. 2009;1164:293–9.

Spiegel R, Kalla R, Rettinger N, Schneider E, Straumann D, Marti S, et al. Head position during resting modifies spontaneous daytime decrease of downbeat nystagmus. Neurology. 2010;75:1928–32.

Strack M, Albrecht H, Pöllmann W, Straube A, Dieterich M. Acquired pendular nystagmus in MS: an examiner-blind cross-over study of memantine and gabapentin. J Neurol. 2010;257:322–7.

Strupp M, Schüler O, Krafczyk S, Jahn K, Schautzer F, Büttner U, et al. Treatment of downbeat-nystagmus with 3,4-diaminopyridine – placebo-controlled study. Neurology. 2003;61:165–70.

Strupp M, Kalla R, Dichgans M, Freilinger T, Glasauer S, Brandt T. Treatment of episodic ataxia type 2 with the potassium channel blocker 4-aminopyridine. Neurology. 2004;62:1623–5.

Strupp M, Versino M, Brandt T. Vestibular migraine. Handb Clin Neurol. 2010;97:755–75.

Strupp M, Kalla R, Claassen J, Adrion C, Mansmann U, Klopstock T, et al. A randomized trial of 4-aminopyridine in EA2 and related familial episodic ataxias. Neurology. 2011a;77:269–75.

Strupp M, Thurtell MJ, Shaikh AS, Brandt T, Zee DS, Leigh RJ. Pharmacotherapy of vestibular and ocular motor disorders, including nystagmus. J Neurol. 2011b;258:1207–22.

Szmulewicz DJ, Waterson JA, Halamgyi GM, Mossmann S, Chancellor AM, McLean CA, et al. Sensory neuropathy as part of the cerebellar ataxia neuropathy vestibular areflexia syndrome. Neurology. 2011;76:1903–10.

Thurtell MJ, Joshi AC, Leone AC, Tomsak RL, Kosmorsky GS, Stahl JS, et al. Cross over-trail of gabapentin and memantine as treatment for acquired nystagmus. Ann Neurol. 2010;67: 676–80.

Tiliket C, Ventre-Dominey J, Vighetto A, Grochowicki M. Room tilt illusion. A central otolith dysfunction. Arch Neurol. 1996;53:1259–64.

Tiliket C, Milea D, Pierrot-Deseilligny C. Upbeat nystagmus from a demyelinating lesion in the caudal pons. J Neuroophthalmol. 2008;28:202–6.

Tsunemi T, Ishikawa K, Tsukui K, Sumi T, Kitamura K, Mizusawa H. The effect of 3,4-diaminopyridine on the patients with hereditary pure cerebellar ataxia. J Neurol Sci. 2010;292:81–4.

Von Brevern M, Zeise D, Neuhauser H, Clarke AH, Lempert T. Acute migrainous vertigo: clinical and oculographic findings. Brain. 2005;128:365–74.

Wagner JN, Glaser M, Brandt T, Strupp M. Downbeat nystagmus: aetiology and comorbidity in 117 patients. J Neurol Neurosurg Psychiatry. 2008;79:672–7.

Weiller C, May A, Limmroth V, Jüpter M, Kaube H, van Schayck R, et al. Brain stem activation in spontaneous human migraine attacks. Nat Med. 1995;1:658–60.

Zee DS, Yamazaki A, Butler PH, Gücer F. Effects of ablation of flocculus and paraflocculus on eye movements in primate. J Neurophysiol. 1981;46:878–99.

zu Eulenburg P, Caspers S, Roski C, Eickhoff SB. Meta-analytical definition and functional connectivity of the human vestibular cortex. Neuroimage. 2012;60:162–9.

Zwergal A, Büttner-Ennever J, Brandt T, Strupp M. An ipsilateral vestibulothalamic tract adjacent to the medial lemniscus in humans. Brain. 2008;131:2928–35.

Chapter 4
Traumatic Forms of Vertigo

4.1 Introduction

After head and neck pain, dizziness is the most frequent chronic complication of a mild head trauma (Friedman 2004; Kashluba et al. 2006; Schütze et al. 2008) or of a whiplash injury. If radiological methods do not reveal a petrous bone fracture with hemotympanum or the presence of air in the labyrinth (pneumolabyrinth) or a brainstem contusion cannot be clinically confirmed, the first questions to ask are the following:

- Is this dizziness organic or psychogenic (Staab 2012)?
- What is the underlying mechanism of the dizziness (peripheral or central vestibular)?

The following posttraumatic forms of vertigo are well known:

- BPPV
- Posttraumatic otolithic vertigo
- Unilateral or bilateral peripheral vestibular disorder culminating in labyrinthine failure (e.g., due to a labyrinth contusion or a petrous bone fracture)
- Perilymph fistula (that leads to a pathological transfer of pressure)
- A barotrauma-induced vertigo.

Frequently a false diagnosis of "cervicogenic vertigo" is made to explain the attacks of dizziness following a whiplash injury. It is still a subject of controversy whether this form of vertigo exists at all and if so, what its pathomechanism could be (see below). However, it is probable that in many cases of a whiplash injury or head trauma, a loosening of otoconia (even without BPPV) takes place, resulting in a posttraumatic otolithic vertigo in the form of a transient gait and postural instability.

T. Brandt et al., *Vertigo and Dizziness*,
DOI 10.1007/978-0-85729-591-0_4, © Springer-Verlag London 2013

4.2   Traumatic Peripheral Vestibular Forms of Vertigo

4.2.1   Posttraumatic BPPV

The most frequent peripheral labyrinthine form of vertigo is BPPV (Sect. 2.2) (http://extra.springer.com).

It is characterized by short attacks of rotatory vertigo and typical rotatory crescendo–decrescendo nystagmus, which is triggered by positioning the head toward the affected ear or tilting it backward and resolves within seconds. Rotatory vertigo and nystagmus occur after positioning with a short latency of seconds and cease temporarily after repeated positioning maneuvers. BPPV occurs in approximately 10 % of patients as posttraumatic positioning vertigo (Gordon et al. 2004; Motin et al. 2005). It is frequently bilateral and asymmetrical (ca. 20 %) and is occasionally also found in children. In two-thirds of the cases, the posterior canal is affected, in one-third, the horizontal canal (Ahn et al. 2011). In our experience the interval between the actual head trauma or whiplash injury and its manifestation as positioning vertigo can last from days up to several weeks. It is possible that the otoconia become detached from the macula bed in two steps or in the first phase remain in the endolymphatic space of the utricle and only reach the canal later, at which time they induce the typical positioning vertigo. This delay can be important in situations requiring expert witness evidence. Immediately after the trauma the patients occasionally complain of unsteadiness of gait (like walking on a mattress), probably due to an "otolithic vertigo." Only subsequently do the typical symptoms of BPPV appear. Traumatic BPPV has been frequently reported after neurosurgical, maxillary, as well as ENT operations of the skull (Chiarella et al. 2007).

The pathophysiology and treatment of posttraumatic BPPV correspond to that of idiopathic BPPV (Sect. 2.2). The therapy phase is occasionally longer, in part because it frequently occurs bilaterally, and liberatory maneuvers have to be repeated, beginning with the treatment of the more-affected ear until the patient is symptom-free (Ahn et al. 2011). The recurrence rate of traumatic BPPV is evidently not higher than that of idiopathic BPPV (Ahn et al. 2011; Brandt et al. 2006, 2010). The different types of liberatory maneuvers (Semont, Epley) are successfully used for a canalolithiasis of the posterior canal (Herdman 1990; Fife et al. 2008). Generally more than 90 % of patients are asymptomatic after 1 week of treatment (von Brevern et al. 2006; Mandala et al. 2012). Cases of the more rarely affected horizontal canal are treated with a "barbecue" maneuver, a 12-h period of lying on the healthy ear (Fife et al. 2008) or by the Gufoni maneuver (Kim et al. 2012). Therapy failures are very rare (<1 %).

4.2.2   Traumatic Labyrinthine Failure

A unilateral hemorrhage or a petrous bone fracture (vestibulocochlear disorders occur more frequently with transverse than with longitudinal fractures) can lead to direct injury of the vestibular nerve or the labyrinth (Sect. 2.2). This causes:

• Violent rotatory vertigo, which continues for days
• Horizontal rotatory nystagmus to the unaffected side

Fig. 4.1 Longitudinal petrous bone fracture: CT of base of skull in bone kernel, two consecutive slices (**a, b**). *Short arrow*: fracture line through the right petrous bone with multiple mastoid cell opacity. *Dashed arrow*: additional fracture of the squamous portion of the right temporal bone (Figure was kindly provided by PD Dr. Jenny Linn, Department of Neuroradiology, University of Munich, Grosshadern)

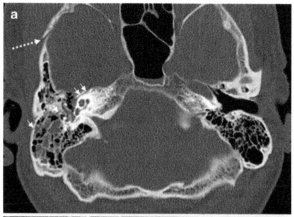
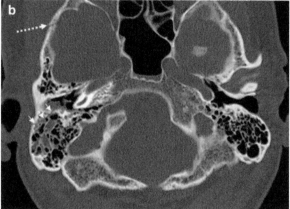

- Posture and gait instability with deviation to the affected side
- Nausea and vomiting.

The clinical symptoms are similar to those of vestibular neuritis (http://extra. springer.com) (Sect. 2.2). Three forms of petrous bone fractures can be differentiated as the following: mixed, longitudinal, and transverse (Rafferty et al. 2006; Gladwell and Viozzi 2008).

- Longitudinal petrous bone fractures (Fig. 4.1) are more frequent; they cause injury to the middle ear and bleeding from the ear.
- The transverse petrous bone fracture with labyrinthine lesion and resulting rotatory vertigo and hearing loss, as well as possible injury to the facial nerve, occur more seldom.

If there is a direct trauma of the petrous bone and corresponding symptoms of rotatory vertigo and hearing loss, but the injury cannot be confirmed either macroscopically or by X-ray, one speaks of a labyrinthine contusion.

The first phase of manifest dysfunction is characterized by a strong feeling of illness with continuous rotatory vertigo, nausea, and vomiting. These symptoms slowly dissipate over 2–3 weeks. Bed rest and antivertiginous drugs (e.g., dimenhydrinate) should be prescribed only within the first days for severe nausea and vomiting. The same limited therapy is recommended for vestibular neuritis, as these drugs delay central compensation. The patient should begin a vestibular training program as soon as possible to accelerate and improve central compensation (Strupp et al. 1998). Similarly, treatment with corticosteroids (methylprednisolone) is also indicated for a few days, in most cases because of trauma-induced edema.

Vertigo, oscillopsia, and hearing loss are also frequent complications of traumas due to military or terrorist blasts (Scherer et al. 2007). They can take a progressive course (Hoffer et al. 2010).

4.2.3   Traumatic Perilymph Fistula

Usually the air in the middle ear is of normal atmospheric pressure, since air supply via the nasopharynx passes through the Eustachian tube. In disorders of air supply to the Eustachian tube, painful pressure gradients occur on the eardrum and in the middle ear. During head trauma, extreme increases in pressure can occur in the middle ear and cause a defect at the round and oval windows or more seldom a luxation of the stapes footplate in the direction of the inner ear with pathological transfer of pressure to the perilymphatic space or with a pneumolabyrinth (Sarac et al. 2006; Hatano et al. 2009). The changes in pressure can also lead to a dehiscence of the anterior semicircular canal (superior canal dehiscence syndrome, Sect. 2.7). The consequences are:

- Attacks of dizziness, in part with oscillopsia (generally due to pressure changes from coughing, pressing, sneezing, lifting heavy weights, or loud sounds)
- Fluctuating hearing loss, seldom autophonia
- Ear pressure
- Tinnitus.

The complaints can depend on the position of the head or on movement as in perilymph fistulas of other etiologies (Maitland 2001; Bourgeois et al. 2005) (Sect. 2.7) (http://extra.springer.com). Generally a high-resolution CT of the inner ear can prove the etiology, e.g., a bony defect of the superior canal. The presence of air in the labyrinth (pneumolabyrinth) following a trauma indicates a traumatic perilymph fistula (Tsubota et al. 2009).

Clinically, dizziness can be classified as either a canal type with rotatory vertigo and nystagmus or an otolithic type (in cases of fistulas of the oval window) with postural vertigo, unsteadiness, and stance and gait ataxia, especially during linear head acceleration (when standing up or walking). The otolithic type of dizziness can also be caused by luxation of the stapes footplate without resulting in continuous perilymph leakage; this happens when the luxated stapes footplate via the peri/endolymph fluid pressure stimulates the otoliths during the acoustically induced stapedial reflex (otolithic Tullio phenomenon). At the same time, loud sounds of certain frequencies induce paroxysmal excitations of the anterior canal in cases of bony dehiscence or otolithic symptoms (head tilt and postural instability).

An initially conservative therapy of several days of bed rest with the head elevated, perhaps mild sedation, and the administration of laxatives results in recovery in the majority of cases. If such conservative therapy fails, and hearing loss or vestibular symptoms increase, then an exploratory tympanotomy or in cases of a dehiscence of the superior canal, surgical canal plugging is indicated.

4.2.4 Alternobaric Vertigo

Rapid changes of pressure in the middle ear— primarily during the decompression experienced by divers (Klingmann et al. 2006) or by pilots and aircrews during flights (Subtil et al. 2007)—can cause a transient rotatory vertigo that is called alternobaric vertigo. At the very beginning of the rotatory vertigo and nystagmus, which spontaneously resolves after seconds or hours, there is a feeling of fullness in the ear. Acute rotatory vertigo indicates an inadequate stimulation of a semicircular canal, which is triggered by an asymmetrical, excessive acute pressure on the round and oval windows in the middle ear (Molvaer and Albrektsen 1988). The same mechanism underlies perilymph fistulas.

Dysfunctions of the Eustachian tube are a special risk factor for developing an alternobaric vertigo (Uzun 2005). Women appear to be at a higher risk of developing alternobaric vertigo during scuba diving than men (Klingmann et al. 2006), but retrospective studies do not show that this vertigo leads to life-threatening situations underwater.

4.2.5 Otolithic Vertigo

Traumatic otolithic vertigo probably occurs more often than is generally assumed (Brandt and Daroff 1980; Ernst et al. 2005). Immediately after a head trauma or after a latency, patients often report having experienced:

- Postural imbalance that is exacerbated by head movements
- Oscillopsia during head movements
- Gait instability that is like walking on a water pillow.

These are typical disorders of otolithic function. As shown in animal studies, the traumatic accelerations probably cause loosening of the otoconia, which leads to unequal otolithic masses on the two sides. The different otolithic weights on the two sides can result in a temporary disturbance of spatial orientation. Within days or weeks, however, central compensation corrects for the otolithic imbalance, and the postural instability during head movements and gait ataxia abates. If complaints persist, a differential diagnosis must be made which takes into account the possibility of a secondary somatoform vertigo.

4.3   Traumatic Central Vestibular Forms of Vertigo

The various central vestibular syndromes are triggered by disorders of brainstem or cerebellar function in connection with a contusion or hemorrhage or, indirectly, due to a traumatic vertebral dissection. In principle, parts of the brainstem and cerebellum, the midbrain and thalamus, the pons to the medulla oblongata and cerebellum, can be affected; the mesencephalon is affected relatively often.

The individual syndromes are described in Sect. 3.1.

4.4   Traumatic Cervicogenic Vertigo

The question of whether there is a medical entity "cervicogenic vertigo" is still a subject of controversy (see Sect. 6.3). The neck afferents not only take part in coordinating eyes, head, and body but they are also involved in the orientation of the body in space and the control of posture. This means that in principle, a stimulation or lesion of these structures could trigger vertigo. It has been shown in animal experiments in primates (*Macaca*) that a unilateral local anesthesia or section of the superior cervical roots induces a tendency to fall due to a temporary increase of tonus of the extensor muscles on the ipsilateral side and a decrease on the contralateral side, as well as ipsiversive past-pointing. Positional nystagmus, however, is elicited only in certain species and to different degrees (most pronounced in rabbits, less in cats) but not at all in Rhesus monkeys (De Jong et al. 1977). This type of positional nystagmus that derives from an imbalance in tonus of the superior cervical roots has not been proven to exist in humans. Patients with C2 root blockades (for cervicogenic headache) exhibit a slight instability of gait with minor ipsilateral deviation of gait and past-pointing without ocular motor disorders (Dieterich et al. 1993); this corresponds to findings in the animal experiments with *Macaca*. One would expect similar symptoms such as instability of gait in "cervicogenic vertigo" always in connection with cervico-vertebrogenic pain and movement restriction of the cervical vertebrae but not with rotatory vertigo or spontaneous, positional, or provocation-induced nystagmus.

Unfortunately, there are still no useful tests to confirm "cervicogenic vertigo" (gait instability), as the tests available use passive head turns while the trunk is fixed and trigger the same amount of nystagmus with the same frequency in healthy subjects (Holtmann et al. 1993). These tests are still in use in some places nowadays, but they fail to give meaningful results. For this reason the differential diagnosis must always include careful otoneurological diagnostics (Ernst et al. 2005), especially if complaints are not initially present but appear only in the course of the disorder. In such a case, a secondary (psychogenic) somatoform vertigo must be considered, since it can appear in up to ca. 50 % of patients with a primarily organic vertigo syndrome, depending on the comorbidity (Eckhardt-Henn et al. 2008).

4.5   Posttraumatic Psychogenic Vertigo

If vertigo persists for a long time after a head trauma or a whiplash injury and otoneurological or ocular motor deficits cannot be determined, this can indicate a psychogenic or somatoform vertigo (Sect. 5).

The most frequent psychosomatic form of vertigo and the second most frequent cause of vertigo in neurological patients is the somatoform phobic postural vertigo (Sect. 5.2). It often occurs secondary to organic forms of vertigo (Huppert et al. 1995; Eckhardt-Henn et al. 2008). A clear increase in the cases of somatoform phobic postural vertigo was observed in Georgia after a strong earthquake (Tevzadze and Shakarishvili 2007). In cases of chronic, long-term complaints, the desire to retire must also be considered in the differential diagnosis.

References

Ahn SK, Jeon SY, Kim JP, Park JJ, Hur DG, Kim DW, et al. Clinical characteristics and treatment of benign paroxysmal positional vertigo after traumatic brain injury. J Trauma. 2011;70: 442–6.

Bourgeois B, Ferron C, Bordure P, Beauvillain de Montreuil C, Legent F. Exploratory tympanotomy for suspected traumatic perilymphatic fistula. Ann Otolaryngol Chir Cervicofac. 2005;122:181–6.

Brandt T, Daroff RB. The multisensory physiological and pathological vertigo syndromes. Ann Neurol. 1980;7:195–203.

Brandt T, Huppert D, Hecht J, Karch C, Strupp M. Benign paroxysmal positioning vertigo: a long-term follow up (6:17 years) of 125 patients. Acta Otolaryngol. 2006;126:160–3.

Brandt T, Huppert D, Hüfner K, Zingler VC, Dieterich M, Strupp M. Long-term course and relapses of vestibular and balance disorders. Rest Neurol Neurosci. 2010;28:69–82.

Chiarella G, Leopardi G, De Fazio L, Chiarella R, Cassandro C, Cassandro E. Iatrogenic benign paroxysmal positional vertigo: review and personal experience in dental and maxillo-facial surgery. Acta Otorhinolaryngol Ital. 2007;27:126–8.

De Jong PTVM, de Jong JMBV, Cohen D, Jongkees LDW. Ataxia and nystagmus induced by injection of local anaesthetics in the neck. Ann Neurol. 1977;1:240–6.

Dieterich M, Pöllmann W, Pfaffenrath V. Cervicogenic headache: electronystagmography, perception of verticality, and posturography in patients before and after C2-blockade. Cephalalgia. 1993;13:285–8.

Eckhardt-Henn A, Best C, Bense S, Breuer P, Diener G, Tschan R, et al. Psychiatric comorbidity in different organic vertigo syndromes. J Neurol. 2008;255:420–8.

Ernst A, Basta D, Seidl RO, Todt I, Scherer H, Clarke A. Management of posttraumatic vertigo. Otolaryngol Head Neck Surg. 2005;132:554–8.

Fife TD, Iverson DJ, Lempert T, Furman JM, Baloh RW, Tusa RJ, et al. Practice parameter: therapies for benign paroxysmal positional vertigo (an evidence-based review): Report of the Quality Standards Subcommittee of the American Academy of Neurology. Neurology. 2008;70: 2067–74.

Friedman JM. Post-traumatic vertigo. Med Health. 2004;87:296–300.

Gladwell M, Viozzi C. Temporal bone fractures: a review for the oral and maxillofacial surgeon. J Oral Maxillofac Surg. 2008;66:513–22.

Gordon CR, Levite R, Joffe V, Gadoth N. Is posttraumatic benign paroxysmal positional vertigo different from the idiopathic form? Arch Neurol. 2004;61:1590–3.

Hatano A, Rikitake M, Komori M, Irie T, Moriyama H. Traumatic perilymph fistula with the luxation of the stapes into the vestibule. Auris Nasus Larynx. 2009;36:474–8.

Herdman S. Treatment of benign paroxysmal positional vertigo. Phys Ther. 1990;6:381–8.

Hoffer ME, Balaban C, Gottshall K, Balough BJ, Maddox MR, Penta JR. Blast exposure: vestibular consequences and associated characteristics. Otol Neurotol. 2010;31:232–6.

Holtmann S, Reiman V, Schöps P. Clinical significance of cervico-ocular reactions. Laryngorhinootologie. 1993;72:306–10.

Huppert D, Kunihiro T, Brandt T. Phobic postural vertigo (154 patients): its association with vestibular disorders. J Audiol. 1995;4:97–103.

Jäger L, Strupp M, Brandt T, Reiser M. Bildgebung von Labyrinth und Nervus vestibularis. Nervenarzt. 1997;68:443–58.

Kashluba S, Casey JE, Paniak C. Evaluating the utility of ICD-10 diagnostic criteria for postconcussion syndrome following mild traumatic brain injury. J Int Neuropsychol Soc. 2006;12:111–8.

Kim JS, Oh SY, Lee SH, Kang JH, Kim DV, Jeong SH, et al. Randomized clinical trial for apogeotropic horizontal canal benign paroxysmal positional vertigo. Neurology. 2012;78:159–66.

Klingmann C, Knauth M, Praetorius M, Plinkert PK. Alternobaric vertigo – really a hazard? Otol Neurotol. 2006;27:1120–5.

Maitland CG. Perilymphatic fistula. Curr Neurol Neurosci Rep. 2001;1:486–1491.

Mandala M, Santoro GP, Asprella Libonati G, Casani AP, Faralli M, Giannoni B, et al. Double-blind randomized trial on short-term efficacy of the Semont maneuver for the treatment of posterior canal benign paroxysmal positional vertigo. J Neurol. 2012;259:882–5.

Molvaer OI, Albrektsen G. Alternobaric vertigo in professional divers. Undersea Biomed Res. 1988;15:271–82.

Motin M, Keren O, Groswasser Z, Gordon CR. Benign paroxysmal positional vertigo as the cause of dizziness in patients after severe traumatic brain injury: diagnosis and treatment. Brain Inj. 2005;19:693–7.

Rafferty MA, McConn Walsh R, Walsh MA. A comparison of temporal bone fracture classification systems. Clin Otolaryngol. 2006;31:287–91.

Sarac S, Cengel S, Sennaroglu L. Pneumolabyrinth following traumatic luxation of the stapes into the vestibule. Int J Pediatr Otorhinolaryngol. 2006;70:159–61.

Scherer M, Burrows H, Pinto R, Somrack E. Characterizing self-reported dizziness and otovestibular impairment among blast-injured traumatic amputees: a pilot study. Mil Med. 2007;172: 731–7.

Schütze M, Kundt G, Buchholz K, Piek J. Which factors are predictive for long-term complaints after mild traumatic brain injuries? Versicherungsmedizin. 2008;60:78–83.

Staab JP. Chronic subjective dizziness. Continuum (Minneap Minn). 2012;18:1118–41.

Strupp M, Arbusow V, Maag KP, Gall C, Brandt T. Vestibular exercises improve central vestibulospinal compensation after vestibular neuritis. Neurology. 1998;51:838–44.

Subtil J, Varandas J, Galrão F, Dos Santos A. Alternobaric vertigo: prevalence in Portuguese Air Force pilots. Acta Otolaryngol. 2007;127:843–6.

Tevzadze N, Shakarishvili R. Vertigo syndromes associated with earthquake in Georgia. Georgian Med News. 2007;148–149:36–9.

Tsubota M, Shojaku H, Watanabe Y. Prognosis of inner ear function in pneumolabyrinth: case report and literature review. Am J Otolaryngol. 2009;30:423–6.

Uzun C. Evaluation of predive parameters related to eustachian tube dysfunction for symptomatic middle ear barotrauma in divers. Otol Neurotol. 2005;26:59–64.

Von Brevern M, Seelig T, Radtke A, Tiel-Wilck K, Neuhauser H. Long-term efficacy of Epley's manoeuvre: a double-blind randomized trial. J Neurol Neurosurg Psychiatry. 2006;77:980–2.

Chapter 5
Somatoform Vertigo and Dizziness Syndromes

5.1 Overview of the Somatoform Vertigo and Dizziness Syndromes

Somatoform vertigo and dizziness account for a large proportion of the complex forms of vertigo syndromes (somatoform is the actual term for "psychogenic"). Two forms are differentiated:

- Primary somatoform vertigo syndromes
- Secondary somatoform vertigo syndromes that develop after vestibular vertigo (Huppert et al. 1995; Dieterich and Eckhardt-Henn 2006; Eckhardt-Henn et al. 2008) (Fig. 5.1)

In the course of their complex somatoform vertigo syndromes, about 70 % of these patients still complain about symptoms, even after several years, and are more impaired in their professional and daily activities than patients with organic forms of dizziness (Furman and Jacob 1997; Yardley and Redfern 2001; Eckhardt-Henn et al. 2003). The most frequent underlying patterns of psychiatric disorders are:

- Anxiety and phobic disorders
- Depressive disorders
- Dissociative disorders (conversion syndrome)
- Somatoform disorders (ICD-10:F45)
- More seldom depersonalization/derealization syndromes

5.1.1 Frequency

There is a high comorbidity between these psychiatric disorders and several organic vertigo syndromes. Structured interviews and various psychometric tests have found evidence of a psychiatric comorbidity of up to 65 % in patients with vestibular migraine and one of 57 % in patients with Menière's disease. In contrast,

T. Brandt et al., *Vertigo and Dizziness*,
DOI 10.1007/978-0-85729-591-0_5, © Springer-Verlag London 2013

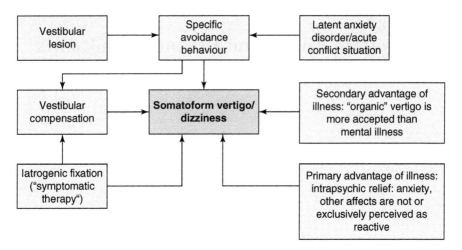

Fig. 5.1 Pathogenetic model: secondary somatoform vertigo/dizziness, triggered by organic vertigo (modified from Dieterich and Eckhardt-Henn (2006))

the comorbidity in patients with BPPV amounts to only 15 % and in patients with vestibular neuritis to 22 %, which approximates the level of 20 % found in normal control groups (Eckhardt-Henn et al. 2008).

Similar findings for psychiatric morbidity and comorbidity have also been reported in a prospective psychometric follow-up study conducted over 1 year in different groups of patients with vestibular vertigo syndromes. While the patients with BPPV, vestibular neuritis, and Menière's disease exhibited normal or normalizing values, it was conspicuous that only the patients with vestibular migraine had a persistent, clearly elevated incidence of psychiatric disorders (Best et al. 2008a; Fig. 5.2). They also felt themselves more hindered in their daily life by dizziness, experienced the vestibular symptoms as being stronger, and had more anxiety than all other vertigo patients (Best et al. 2009b; Tschan et al. 2011). Moreover, patients with a prehistory of a mental illness were at a clearly higher risk of becoming ill with another psychiatric disorder following a vestibular vertigo syndrome (Fig. 5.3). However, the extent of vestibular injury or vestibular dysfunction had no influence on the further course of the psychiatric stress (Best et al. 2006, 2009a, b).

Only the degree of the initially experienced vertigo, not that of the vestibular function disorder, had a predictive value in patients with vestibular neuritis, but not in patients with BPPV for the development of a somatoform vertigo in the course of the disorder (Heinrichs et al. 2007). Even a persistent anxiety about a renewed episode of vertigo had predictive value for the later occurrence of a panic or somatoform disorder in patients with vestibular neuritis (Godemann et al. 2006).

Since primarily patients with vestibular migraine are at a particularly high risk of developing a somatoform vertigo, this possibility should be considered early in the therapeutic deliberations.

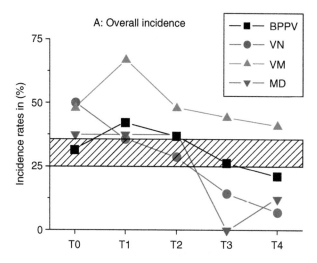

Fig. 5.2 Prospective longitudinal analysis of the incidence (in %) of the development of a soma-toform/psychiatric disorder in the course of illness in patients with various vestibular vertigo syn-dromes. Patients with vestibular migraine develop a secondary somatoform disorder conspicuously more often (*BPPV* benign peripheral paroxysmal positioning vertigo, *VN* vestibular neuritis, *VM* vestibular migraine, *MD* Menière's disease, *T0* time of the diagnosis of the illness, *T1* 6 weeks, *T2* 3 months, *T3* 6 months, *T4* 1 year)

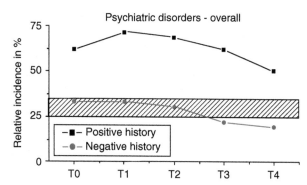

Fig. 5.3 Relative incidence of a patient becoming ill with a psychiatric disorder after having had a vestibular vertigo syndrome dependent on his/her prehistory of psychiatric disorders

5.1.2   Patient History

Since somatoform dizziness first seems to occur without psychopathological symptoms, as a rule this causes the patients to go to ENT doctors, neurologists, or internists. The patients describe experiencing frequent (http://extra.springer.com):

- Postural imbalance or a diffuse feeling of dizziness
- Light-headedness
- An emptiness in the head
- Unsteadiness when walking

- A feeling of toppling over or of losing touch with the ground
- Very rarely rotatory vertigo with accompanying vegetative symptoms and nausea

Depending on the underlying psychiatric disease (see above), the following additional symptoms can be present:

- Disorders of motivation and concentration
- Decline in performance
- Subjectively experienced restrictions in professional and daily activities
- Vegetative symptoms that accompany the dizziness (accelerated heart rate, nausea, sweats, apnea, fear of suffocating, loss of appetite, weight loss)
- Emotional and mood disorders
- Sleep disturbances
- Symptoms of anxiety

Typically all of these symptoms are experienced and described as reactive, i.e., the patients believe that the symptoms are triggered and induced by the dizziness. Patients seldom spontaneously report conflict and stress situations that can function as triggers of vertigo/dizziness; often they are initially totally unaware of them. This makes it difficult to establish the diagnosis.

5.1.3 Pathophysiology and Therapeutic Principles

Currently two pathogenetic mechanisms of somatoform vertigo are differentiated:

- *Primary somatoform vertigo syndromes* that occur without preceding organic vertigo syndromes and have similar pathogenetic mechanisms like those of the underlying psychiatric disorders (anxiety or phobic, depressive, dissociative, or somatoform disorders)
- *Secondary somatoform vertigo syndromes* that occur during or after an organic vertigo syndrome

In certain predisposed patients a feedback loop between a bodily sensation (e.g., light-headedness) or a physical symptom of illness (e.g., rotatory vertigo in vestibular neuritis) results in a cognitive-catastrophizing interpretation, i.e., the bodily symptom is seen as a danger, as an expression of a basically severe or life-threatening physical illness. Subsequently anxiety and panic reactions can escalate in intensity. Such somatosensory amplification is an established model of somatoform disorders (Barsky and Wyshak 1990).

The treatment depends on the clinical picture and on the exact classification by the psychiatrist/psychosomatician of the somatoform syndromes (anxiety and phobic disorder, depression, dissociative, or somatoform disorder). The degree and the chronification of the syndrome should determine when psychotherapy and/or pharmacotherapy is begun. Since good prospective studies are not yet available, it cannot be decided which therapy is most suitable for which form of somatoform vertigo/dizziness. A pilot study recently gave first indications that a cognitive behavioural therapeutic training program can reduce the dysfunctional aspect of the illness and the dizziness (Tschan et al. 2012). A systematic analysis of previous therapy studies was able to prove the efficacy of psychotherapeutic–psychosomatic treatment approaches (Schmid et al. 2011).

The indication for therapy depends on the clinical findings and the underlying conflict or stress situation. Outpatient therapy focusing on the leading symptom can be quite successful in cases of short-term dizziness that is not very pronounced. Long-term techniques should be selected according to the underlying conflict situation (e.g., psychodynamic therapy or psychoanalysis). For subjects with a strongly pronounced disorder and considerable suffering, we recommend a combination therapy with a psychoactive drug; the drugs of choice belong to the scrotonin reuptake inhibitors. In a few patients it is necessary to initially combine these drugs with an anxiolytic drug for a short time.

5.2 Phobic Postural Vertigo

In the following, phobic postural vertigo, an important and the most frequent form of somatoform vertigo/dizziness, is discussed in detail.

5.2.1 Patient History

The cardinal symptoms and features of phobic postural vertigo include the following (Brandt and Dieterich 1986; Brandt 1996):

- Patients complain about postural dizziness and subjective stance and gait unsteadiness without this being evident to an observer; moreover, their findings in neuro-otological tests are normal.
- Dizziness is often described as light-headedness with varying degrees of unsteadiness of stance and gait, attack-like fear of falling without any real falls, in part also unintentional body swaying of short duration.
- The attacks often occur in typical situations known to be external triggers of other phobic syndromes (e.g., bridges, driving a car, empty rooms, long corridors, large crowds of people in a store or restaurant) or during visual stimulation (e.g., cinema, television, store).
- Vertigo improves or resolves during sport activities (bicycling, tennis) and during more complicated balance conditions, whereas it appears again at rest or under simpler conditions (e.g., standing after bicycling).
- During the course of the illness, the patient begins to generalize the symptoms and increasingly to avoid the triggering stimuli. During or shortly after the attacks (frequently mentioned only when asked), patients report vegetative disturbances and anxiety; most also report attacks of vertigo/dizziness without anxiety.

- If asked, patients usually report that their symptoms improve after imbibing a little alcohol.
- Initially there is often an organic vestibular illness, e.g., resolved vestibular neuritis, BPPV (Huppert et al. 1995), or special psychosocial stress situations (Kapfhammer et al. 1997).
- Patients with phobic postural vertigo often exhibit obsessive–compulsive and perfectionistic personality traits and reactive–depressive symptoms during the course of the disease.

Here it is important to determine these so-called "positive" criteria of the symptoms and not only exclude other illnesses.

5.2.2 Clinical Aspects and Course of the Illness

The combination of postural vertigo with subjective instability of stance and gait in patients with normal neurological findings in vestibular and balance test results (otoneurological examination, video-oculography including caloric irrigation, imaging) or disorders that cannot explain the symptoms and a compulsive personality structure are characteristic. The monosymptomatic subjective disorder of balance is connected with standing or walking and manifests with attack-like worsening that occurs with or without recognizable triggers and with or without accompanying anxiety. The absence of recognizable triggers or vertigo without accompanying anxiety causes many patients and occasionally the doctor treating them to doubt the diagnosis of a somatoform disorder.

Patients with phobic postural vertigo generally have a compulsive primary personality (in the sense of "pronounced personality traits") and a tendency to intensified introspection and the need "to keep everything under control." They are more likely to be ambitious and place high demands on themselves and are often easily irritated and fearful.

Such patients rarely go to a psychiatrist first; they tend to see the "specialist" for their symptom, especially as they feel themselves to be organically sick. However, as phobic postural vertigo is not yet part of the diagnostic repertoire of most neurologists and ENT doctors, the illness often lasts quite a long time before a diagnosis is established (an average of 3 years for 154 patients with phobic postural vertigo; Huppert et al. 1995). The diagnosis is established only after a number of visits to different specialists, superfluous laboratory examinations, and erroneous classifications such as "cervicogenic vertigo" or "recurrent vertebrobasilar ischemia," with correspondingly unsuccessful treatment attempts.

Phobic postural vertigo is the most frequent cause of vertigo in younger adults (Strupp et al. 2003). A psychiatric follow-up study confirmed that phobic postural vertigo is a unique medical entity, which can be clearly differentiated from panic disorder with or without agoraphobia (Kapfhammer et al. 1997). Another longitudinal follow-up study (5–16 years) on 106 patients showed an improvement rate of

75 %; the symptoms had fully resolved in 27 % (Huppert et al. 2005). In none of these patients did the diagnosis have to be revised.

Phobic postural vertigo can manifest in adults of every age, most often in the second and fifth decades (it is the most common form of vertigo in this age group), and it shows no sexual predominance (Strupp et al. 2003). If phobic postural vertigo remains untreated, the symptoms worsen, generalization develops, and avoidance behavior increases until the patient is unable to leave his/her own apartment without help.

5.2.3   Pathophysiology and Therapeutic Principles

To explain the illusory perception of postural vertigo and stance instability, we have hypothesized a disturbance of space constancy, which results from a partial decoupling of the actual re-afference from the efference-copy signal for active head and body movements (Brandt and Dieterich 1986; Brandt 1996). Under normal conditions, we do not perceive such slight, self-generated body sway or head movements as accelerations during upright stance. The environment also appears to be stationary during active movements, although there are shifts of retinal images caused by these relative movements. Space constancy seems to be maintained by the simultaneous occurrence of a voluntary impulse to initiate a movement and the delivery of adequate information in parallel to identify self-motion (Fig. 5.4). According to von Holst and Mittelstaedt (1950), this efference copy may provide a sensory pattern of expectation based on earlier experience (internal model), which by means of the movement-triggered actual sensory information is then so interpreted that self-motion can be differentiated from the motion of the environment. If this efference copy is missing, e.g., if we move the eyeball with a finger on the eyelid, illusory movements of the environment occur, so-called oscillopsia. The sensation of vertigo described by these patients (involving involuntary body sway and the occasional perception of individual head movements as disturbing external perturbations with simultaneous illusional movements of the surroundings) can be explained by a transient decoupling of efference copy and re-afference, i.e., a mismatch occurs between the anticipated and the actual motion.

Healthy persons can experience similar mild sensations of vertigo without simultaneous anxiety during a state of total exhaustion, when the difference between voluntary head movements and involuntary sway becomes blurred. In patients with phobic postural vertigo, this partial decoupling may be caused by their constant preoccupation with anxious monitoring and checking of balance. This leads to the perception of sensorimotor adjustments that would otherwise be made unconsciously by means of learned (and reflex-like) muscle activation programs called up to maintain upright posture.

Precise posturographic analyses show that these patients increase their postural sway during normal stance by co-contracting the flexor and extensor muscles of the foot. This is evidently an expression of an unnecessary fearful strategy to

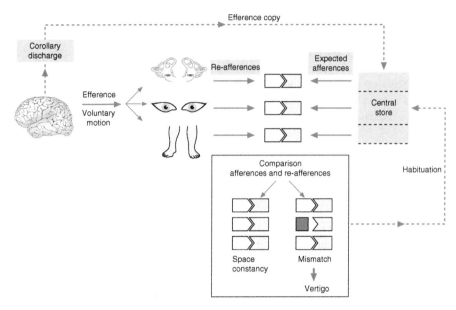

Fig. 5.4 Schematic drawing showing how vertigo/dizziness develops due to a disturbance of the space-constancy mechanism during active motion (modified from Brandt (1996)). Voluntary head movements lead to stimulation of the vestibular, visual, and somatosensory organs. Their messages are compared with a multisensory pattern of expectation provided by an internal model that was calibrated by earlier experience of motion. The expected pattern is prepared simultaneously by the efference-copy signal, which is sent in parallel with the voluntary movement impulse. If the concurrent sensory stimulation and the pattern of expectation are in agreement, the self-motion is perceived and "space constancy" is maintained. However, if there is an incongruence between the incoming and the expected pattern due to a partial "decoupling" of the efference-copy signal and the re-afference, a sensorimotor mismatch, then vertigo and imbalance are perceived. The subject no longer experiences a voluntary head movement in a stationary surrounding but rather a threatening disorientation with exogenic head acceleration and a concurrent illusory movement of the surrounding

control stance. Subjective imbalance in phobic postural vertigo is associated with characteristic changes in the coordination of open- and closed-loop mechanisms of postural control by which sensory feedback is used inadequately during undisturbed stance (Wuehr et al. 2013). Healthy subjects use this strategy only when in real danger of falling. During difficult balancing tasks, such as tandem stance with eyes closed, the posturographic data of the patients do not differ from those of healthy subjects, i.e., the more difficult the demands of balance, the more "healthy" the balance performance of the patients with phobic postural vertigo (Querner et al. 2000; Fig. 5.5). These patients often report that unsteadiness especially increases when looking at moving visual scenes. However, when exposed to large-field visual motion stimulation in the roll plane, body sway did not exhibit any increased risk of falling (Querner et al. 2002). The use of automatized analysis of sway patterns in posturography (Sect. 1.7.6) under various conditions (e.g., with eyes open or closed, standing on firm ground or on foam rubber) together with a neuronal network allows in many cases a decision as to whether, for example,

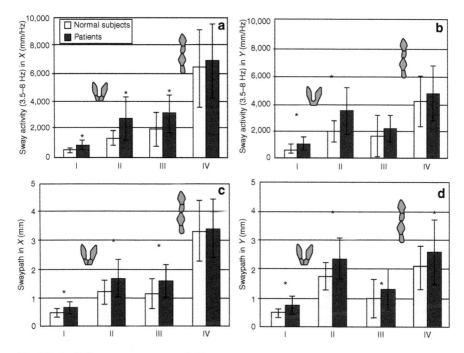

Fig. 5.5 (**a–d**) Sway parameters revealed by a posturographic examination of healthy subjects and patients with phobic postural vertigo during different conditions of stance of increasing difficulty (*I* normal stance with eyes open, *II* normal stance with eyes closed, *III* tandem stance with eyes open, *IV* tandem stance with eyes closed). The more difficult the conditions, the more normal the performance of patients with phobic postural vertigo (modified from Querner et al. (2000))

a phobic postural vertigo is present or other important differential diagnoses (e.g., bilateral vestibulopathy, orthostatic tremor, or cerebellar syndrome) (Krafczyk et al. 2006; Brandt et al. 2012).

A doctor–patient consultation that provides a detailed explanation of the mechanism of the disease and of the necessity of self-controlled desensitization, i.e., the patient should consciously confront situations that induce dizziness, is essential for the therapy to succeed.

5.2.4 Pragmatic Therapy

The treatment is based on three or four measures:

- A thorough diagnosis to convince the patients that the symptoms are not caused by an organic disorder
- "Psychoeducational" explanation
- Desensitization by self-exposure to triggers and regular exercise
- If symptoms persist, behavioral therapy with or without accompanying pharmacotherapy

In our experience, the most important therapeutic measure is to relieve the patient of his fear of having an organic illness by carefully examining him and explaining the psychogenic mechanism ("increased self-observation" in the context of the corresponding primary personality structure). Desensitization by exposure to the causative situations should follow, i.e., the patient should not avoid such situations but, on the contrary, seek them out. At the same time, regular exercise has proven to be helpful to give the patient confidence in his/her own sense of balance. If the explanation and self-desensitization do not result in sufficient improvement after weeks to months, behavioral therapy with or without drug therapy should be started, i.e., with a selective serotonin reuptake inhibitor (e.g., paroxetine, citalopram, fluvoxamine, or sertraline) or a tri-/tetracyclic antidepressive drug for 3–6 months. In a few patients it is necessary to initially combine these drugs with an anxiolytic drug (e.g., lorazepam) but only for a short time because of the danger of addiction.

In a follow-up study (0.5–5.5 years after the initial diagnosis) involving 78 patients, we showed that 72 % of the patients were free of symptoms or exhibited a clear improvement after this therapeutic strategy (Brandt et al. 1994). Fortunately this long-term follow-up study showed no sign of an erroneous diagnosis. Identical results were also found in a long-term follow-up study over 5–16 years (Huppert et al. 2005).

Cognitive and behavioral therapy in combination with vestibular rehabilitation was shown to significantly improve symptoms in controlled studies with small groups of patients (Andersson et al. 2006; Holmberg et al. 2006). However, a follow-up examination after 1 year in a part of the treated patients determined that the positive effect was not maintained (Holmberg et al. 2007). Probably a combination of cognitive and behavioral therapy with drugs and physiotherapy including vestibular training is more suitable (pilot study; Tschan et al. 2012).

The readiness of most of the patients, who experience much stress as a result of their suffering, to understand the psychogenic mechanism and to overcome it by desensitization is a positive experience for both the physician and the patients.

5.2.5   Differential Diagnosis and Clinical Problems

The differential diagnosis of phobic postural vertigo includes psychiatric syndromes as well as vestibular and non-vestibular organic syndromes.

The most important psychiatric syndromes besides the types of somatoform vertigo in anxiety, depression, dissociative, and somatoform disorders in a narrower sense (ICD10: F45) include the following:

- Panic disorder with or without agoraphobia
- Space phobia (Marks 1981)
- Visual vertigo (Bronstein 1995, 2004) or chronic subjective dizziness (Staab 2012) overlaps with phobic postural vertigo
- Mal-de-debarquement syndrome (Murphy 1993)

The most important organic syndromes include:

- Primary orthostatic tremor with a pathognomonic frequency peak of 14–16 Hz in electromyography and posturography (Yarrow et al. 2001)
- Bilateral vestibulopathy
- Vestibular paroxysmia
- Perilymph fistula/superior canal dehiscence syndrome
- Vestibular migraine
- Episodic ataxia type 2
- Neurodegenerative disorders (spinocerebellar ataxias, multisystem atrophy)
- Central vestibular syndromes
- Orthostatic dysregulation

In contrast to the long list of possible differential diagnoses, the combination of traits connected with the complaints, normal physical findings, and primary personality type are so characteristic that there is seldom any doubt as to the diagnosis after the first examination.

References

Andersson G, Asmundson GJ, Denev J, Nilsson J, Larsen HC. A controlled trial of cognitive behavior therapy combined with vestibular rehabilitation in the treatment of dizziness. Behav Res Ther. 2006;44:1265–73.

Barsky AJ, Wyshak GL. Hypochondriasis and somatosensory amplification. Br J Psychiatry. 1990;157:404–9.

Best C, Eckhardt-Henn A, Diener G, Bense S, Breuer P, Dieterich M. Interaction of somatoform and vestibular disorders. J Neurol Neurosurg Psychiatry. 2006;77:658–64.

Best C, Eckhardt-Henn A, Tschan R, Bense S, Dieterich M. Psychiatric morbidity and comorbidity in different vestibular vertigo syndrome: results of a prospective longitudinal study over one year. J Neurol. 2009a;256:58–65.

Best C, Eckhardt-Henn A, Tschan R, Dieterich M. Who is a risk for psychiatric distressed after vestibular disorder? Results from a prospective one-year follow-up. Neuroscience. 2009b;164: 1579–87.

Brandt T. Phobic postural vertigo. Neurology. 1996;46:1515–9.

Brandt T, Dieterich M. Phobischer Attacken-Schwankschwindel, ein neues Syndrom. Munch Med Wochenschr. 1986;128:247–50.

Brandt T, Huppert D, Dieterich M. Phobic postural vertigo: a first follow-up. J Neurol. 1994;241: 191–5.

Brandt T, Strupp M, Novozhilov S, Krafczyk S. Artificial neural network posturography detects the transition of vestibular neuritis to phobic postural vertigo. J Neurol. 2012;259:182–4.

Bronstein AM. The visual vertigo syndrome. Acta Otolaryngol (Stockh). 1995;520:45–8.

Bronstein AM. Vision and vertigo: some visual aspects of vestibular disorders. J Neurol. 2004;251:381–7.

Dieterich M, Eckhardt-Henn A. Neurologische und somatoforme Schwindelsyndrome. In: Henningsen P, Gündel H, Ceballos-Baumann A, editors. Neuro-Psychosomatik. Grundlagen und Klinik neurologischer Psychosomatik. Stuttgart: Schattauer; 2006. p. 253–65.

Eckhardt-Henn A, Breuer P, Thomalske C, Hoffmann SO, Hopf HC. Anxiety disorders and other psychiatric subgroups in patients complaining of dizziness. J Anxiety Disord. 2003;431:1–20.

Eckhardt-Henn A, Best C, Bense S, Breuer P, Diener G, Tschan R, et al. Psychiatric comorbidity in different organic vertigo syndromes. J Neurol. 2008;255:420–8.

Furman JM, Jacob RG. Psychiatric dizziness. Neurology. 1997;48:1161–6.

Godemann F, Schabowska A, Naetebusch B, Heinz A, Ströhle A. The impact of cognitions on the development of panic and somatoform disorders: a prospective study in patients with vestibular neuritis. Psychol Med. 2006;36:99–108.

Heinrichs N, Edler C, Eskens S, Mielczarek MM, Moschner C. Predicting continued dizziness after an acute peripheral vestibular disorder. Psychosom Med. 2007;69:700–7.

Holmberg J, Karlberg M, Harlacher U, Rivano-Fischer M, Magnusson M. Treatment of phobic postural vertigo. A controlled study of cognitive-behavioral therapy and self-controlled desensitization. J Neurol. 2006;253:500–6.

Holmberg J, Karlberg M, Harlacher U, Magnusson M. One-year follow-up of cognitive behavioural therapy for phobic postural vertigo. J Neurol. 2007;254:1189–92.

Huppert D, Kunihiro T, Brandt T. Phobic postural vertigo (154 patients): its association with vestibular disorders. J Audiol. 1995;4:97–103.

Huppert D, Strupp M, Rettinger N, Hecht J, Brandt T. Phobic postural vertigo – a long-term follow-up (5–15 years) of 106 patients. J Neurol. 2005;252:564–9.

Kapfhammer HP, Mayer C, Hock U, Huppert D, Dieterich M, Brandt T. Course of illness in phobic postural vertigo. Acta Neurol Scand. 1997;95:23–8.

Krafczyk S, Tietze S, Swoboda W, Valkovic P, Brandt T. Artificial neural network: a new diagnostic posturographic tool for disorders of stance. Clin Neurophysiol. 2006;117:1692–8.

Marks JM. Space "phobia": a pseudo-agoraphobic syndrome. J Neurol Neurosurg Psychiatry. 1981;48:729–35.

Murphy TP. Mal de debarquement syndrome: a forgotten entity? Otolaryngol Head Neck Surg. 1993;109:10–3.

Querner V, Krafczyk S, Dieterich M, Brandt T. Patients with somatoform phobic postural vertigo: the more difficult the balance task, the better the balance performance. Neurosci Lett. 2000;285:21–4.

Querner V, Krafczyk S, Dieterich M, Brandt T. Somatoform phobic postural vertigo: body sway during optokinetically induced roll vection. Exp Brain Res. 2002;143:269–75.

Schmid G, Henningsen P, Dieterich M, Sattel H, Lahmann C. Psychotherapy in vertigo – a systematic review. J Neurol Neurosurg Psychiatry. 2011;82(6):601–6.

Staab JP. Chronic subjective dizziness. Continuum (Minneap Minn). 2012;18:1118–41.

Strupp M, Glaser M, Karch C, Rettinger N, Dieterich M, Brandt T. The most common form of dizziness in middle age: phobic postural vertigo. Nervenarzt. 2003;74:911–4.

Tschan R, Best C, Beutel M, Knebel A, Wiltink J, Dieterich M, et al. Patients' psychological well-being and resilient coping protect from secondary somatoform vertigo and dizziness (SVD) one year after vestibular disease. J Neurol. 2011;258:104–12.

Tschan R, Eckhardt-Henn A, Scheurich V, Best C, Dieterich M, Beutel M. Steadfast-effectiveness of a cognitive behavioral self-management program of patients with somatoform vertigo and dizziness. Psychother Psychosom Med Psychol. 2012;62(3–4):111–9.

Von Holst E, Mittelstaedt H. Das Reafferenzierungsprinzip (Wechselwirkungen zwischen Zentralnervensystem und Peripherie). Naturwissenschaften. 1950;37:461–76.

Wuehr M, Pradhan C, Novozhilov S, Krafczyk S, Brandt T, Jahn K, Schniepp R. Inadequate interaction between open- and closed-loop postural control in phobic postural vertigo. J Neurol. 2013;260:1314–23.

Yardley L, Redfern MS. Psychological factors influencing recovery from balance disorders. J Anxiety Disord. 2001;15:107–19.

Yarrow K, Brown P, Gresty MA, Bronstein AM. Force platform recordings in the diagnosis of primary orthostatic tremor. Gait Posture. 2001;13:27–34.

Chapter 6
Various Vertigo Syndromes

6.1 Vertigo in Childhood and Hereditary Vertigo Syndromes

Dizziness occurs less often as a major symptom in childhood than in adulthood. The prevalence of dizziness in children of school age (at least one attack of dizziness in the previous year) amounts to about 15 % (Russel and Abu-Arafeh 1999). Most forms of dizziness and vestibular syndromes of adulthood, however, can also occur in childhood. For this reason, we will restrict ourselves in this chapter to the essential features of an indicative patient history. Children describe their complaints—depending on their age—less precisely and with less relevance for therapy than do adults. Moreover, the examination results for balance and ocular motor functions depend more on their concerted cooperation.

Episodic vertigo syndromes in childhood are associated with migraine in about 50 % of the cases (Jahn et al. 2009, 2011), appearing as benign paroxysmal vertigo of childhood (Basser 1964), vestibular migraine, or migraine of the basilar type (Sect. 3.2). An epileptic aura, perilymph fistulas, or episodic ataxias occur more rarely. There is also a unilateral (Lee et al. 2011) or a bilateral (Kanaan et al. 2011) bony dehiscence of the superior semicircular canal syndrome in childhood; it differs from that in adults in manifesting primarily with auditory symptoms (autophonia, tinnitus, and hearing disorders). Initial experience has shown that conservative treatment should be given first (Lee et al. 2011). Sustained rotatory vertigo can be the main symptom of vestibular neuritis, a labyrinthitis, or traumatic brain injury. BPPV in children is also generally caused by trauma. Oscillopsia during head movements and balance disorders that worsen in darkness are typical for bilateral vestibulopathy, which is generally caused in children by labyrinthine malformation, viral inflammations, bacterial meningitis, or ototoxic antibiotics (Table 6.1). Predisposing factors for vertigo in childhood are recurrent bouts of otitis, traumatic brain injury, as well as a positive family history of migraine (Niemensivu et al. 2007).

Children with central vestibular signs that begin subacutely should undergo an MRI examination because of the relative frequency of infratentorial brainstem and cerebellar tumors in childhood (Jahn et al. 2009). The percentage of psychogenic or

Table 6.1 Vertigo and disturbance of vestibular function in childhood

Labyrinth/nerve	Central vestibular origin
Hereditary/congenital	
Labyrinthine malformation	Familial episodic ataxia type II
Perilymph fistulas	Downbeat nystagmus
Embryopathic malformations (rubella, cytomegalovirus)	Upbeat nystagmus
Toxic agents	
Various hereditary audiovestibular syndromes	
Familial vestibular areflexia	
Syphilitic labyrinthitis (endolymphatic hydrops)	
Positive family history of migraine	
Benign paroxysmal vertigo of childhood	
Vestibular migraine, basilar-type migraine	
Acquired	
Labyrinthitis with vestibulopathy (viral, bacterial, tuberculosis)	Infratentorial tumors (medulloblastoma, astrocytoma, epidermoid cysts, meningioma)
Perilymph fistulas	Epileptic aura, vestibular epilepsy
Trauma (transverse petrous bone fracture, benign paroxysmal positioning vertigo)	Trauma (brainstem or vestibulocerebellar concussion)
Menière's disease (endolymphatic hydrops)	Encephalitis
Vestibular neuritis	Toxic agents (e.g., upbeat/downbeat nystagmus when on anticonvulsants)
Herpes zoster oticus	
Cholesteatoma	
Ototoxic drugs	
Cogan's syndrome, other inner-ear autoimmune disorders	

somatoform causes of vertigo in children amounts to 5–10 % (Erbek et al. 2006; Riina et al. 2005).

6.1.1   Therapy of Childhood Forms of Vertigo

The treatment of these various forms of vertigo corresponds to that in adults; however, a pediatrician should be closely consulted (Table 6.2). There are no specific studies available on the therapy of most forms of vertigo in childhood. Consequently, the treatment recommendations are similar to those made for adults but with adjusted dosages.

6.1.2   Differential Diagnoses of Childhood Forms of Vertigo

The following three main symptoms (with or without accompanying clinical findings) are helpful for the differential diagnosis of childhood forms of vertigo.

Table 6.2 Therapy for dizziness in children

Vertigo syndrome	Therapy
Migraine-associated vertigo	
Benign paroxysmal vertigo of childhood (BPV)	• Drug migraine prophylaxis only in frequent and severely impairing attacks (favorable spontaneous course)
Basilar-type migraine	• Avoid triggers
Vestibular migraine	• Relaxation techniques
	• Endurance sports
	• Migraine prophylaxis for many (>3) and severe attacks (>72 h)
	– Propranolol 1–2 mg/kg/day
	– Metoprolol succinate 1 mg/kg/day
	– Flunarizin 5 mg/day
	– Topiramate 1–2 mg/kg/day
	– Amitriptyline 1 mg/kg/day
	– Valproate 10–45 mg/kg/day
	– Levetiracetam 20–40 mg/kg/day
	– Lamotrigin 1 mg/kg/day
	– Magnesium 2 mg/kg/day
Benign peripheral paroxysmal positional vertigo (BPPV)	
Posterior canal (>90 %) or horizontal canal	• Liberatory maneuver (Sect. 2.2)
Motion sickness	• Prophylaxis with visual control of vehicle motion
	• Avoiding heavy meals
	• Sufficient fresh air
	• Prophylaxis with drugs:
	– Dimenhydrinate 1–1.5 mg/kg, if necessary, repeat after 6 h
Acute unilateral labyrinthine deficit	
Labyrinthitis:	• Acute symptomatic therapy
	• Early mobilization (central compensation; see Sect. 2.3)
	• Specific therapy for cause
Viral	*Viral*:
	• In zoster oticus, acyclovir 3×5 mg/kg/day; otherwise symptomatic
Bacterial (in meningitis)	*Bacterial*:
	• Antibiotic according to pathogen
Serous in middle-ear infection	*Serous*:
	• Therapy for middle-ear infection according to pathogen
Autoimmune (e.g., Cogan's syndrome)	*Autoimmune*:
	• Prednisolone 1 mg/kg/day, taper according to course
Vestibular neuritis	*Vestibular neuritis*:
	• Prednisolone 1 mg/kg/day, reduce every third day by 20 %
Menière's disease	• Betahistine (no proof)
Traumatic inner-ear damage (petrous bone fracture)	• Balance training
Vestibular paroxysmia	• Carbamazepine 2–6 mg/kg/day
	• Alternative: oxcarbazepine 4–8 mg/kg/day

(continued)

Table 6.2 (continued)

Vertigo syndrome	Therapy
Perilymph fistula	
External fistula to the middle ear (posttraumatic, post-infectious, cholesteatoma)	• Therapy for underlying illness
Internal fistula to the middle posterior fossa	• Generally conservative; operation seldom necessary
Superior canal dehiscence syndrome (posttraumatic, congenital)	• Therapy initially conservative, surgical plugging of canal in rare cases
Bilateral vestibulopathy	
Congenital	For all: • Balance training with gait training and stimulation of the visual and somatosensory systems by head/body movements
Post-infectious (meningitis)	• Specific therapy according to etiology
Toxic (aminoglycosides) malnutritive (vitamin B12, folic acid)	
Autoimmune	
Degenerative (spinocerebellar ataxia)	
Neoplastic (bilateral vestibular schwannoma)	
Idiopathic	
Central vestibular syndromes	
Neoplastic (Tumor—cerebellar/brainstem)	• Therapy according to etiology – Episodic ataxia type II
Degenerative/hereditary (spinocerebellar ataxias, episodic ataxia)	○ Acetazolamide 5–10 mg/kg/day ○ 4-Aminopyridine 3×5 mg/day (consideration of each individual case, insufficient experience in children)
Inflammatory (brainstem encephalitis)	– Downbeat nystagmus/upbeat nystagmus
Vascular (malformation)	○ 4-Aminopyridine (see above)
Traumatic (brainstem contusion)	○ Gabapentin
Epileptic (vestibular aura)	○ Baclofen
Psychosomatic dizziness	• Clarification
	• Desensibilization in cases of avoidance behavior
	• Behavioral therapy
	• Specific therapy based on psychopathological and psychodynamic findings

Modified from Jahn et al. (2009)

6.1.2.1 Attacks of Vertigo

• *Episodic vertigo without pathological findings in the attack-free interval*: benign paroxysmal vertigo of childhood/vestibular migraine, vestibular paroxysmia, epileptic aura or vestibular epilepsy, orthostatic dysregulation, or psychogenic vertigo

- *Episodic vertigo with inner-ear hypoacusis*: perilymph fistula, superior canal dehiscence syndrome, Menière's disease, and vestibular paroxysmia (http:// extra.springer.com)
- *Episodic vertigo with ocular motor abnormalities in the attack-free interval*: basilar-type or vestibular migraine and familial episodic ataxia type 2
- *Episodic vertigo followed in the course of the disease by oscillopsia during head movements and imbalance that worsens in darkness*: development of bilateral vestibular failure (also with familial vestibulopathy)
- Paroxysmal, short (<1 min) attacks of rotatory vertigo during changes in head position relative to gravity: BPPV (posttraumatic)

6.1.2.2 Sustained Vertigo (Lasting Days or a Few Weeks)

- *Sustained vertigo without hearing loss*: acute vestibular neuritis
- *Sustained vertigo with hearing loss*: labyrinthitis and inner-ear autoimmune disease
- *Posttraumatic sustained vertigo*: transverse petrous bone fracture and labyrinthine concussion

6.1.2.3 Stance and Gait Imbalance with and Without Oscillopsia

- *Delayed stance and gait development with or without hearing loss*: congenital bilateral vestibulopathy
- *Stance and gait instability with oscillopsia during walking and head movements*: congenital or early acquired bilateral vestibulopathy, perilymph fistula, and posttraumatic otolithic vertigo
- *Slowly increasing stance and gait instability as well as oscillopsia during head movements*: various hereditary and congenital disorders causing progressive audiovestibular loss
- *Progressive ataxia, balance, and ocular motor disorders*: infratentorial tumors with lesions of vestibulocerebellar and/or pontomedullary brainstem structures and spinocerebellar ataxias with or without downbeat nystagmus.

We now discuss in detail three special forms of vestibular syndromes in childhood.

6.1.3 Benign Paroxysmal Vertigo of Childhood

Benign paroxysmal vertigo of childhood—a vestibular migraine with aura but without headache—is not rare; it is probably the most frequent form of episodic vertigo in childhood. It has a prevalence of 2.6 % (Abu-Arafeh and Russel 1995) and is characterized by sudden brief attacks of vertigo associated with nystagmus. It normally begins between ages 1 and 4 years and remits spontaneously within a few years. The course of the disease is, however, not homogeneous. In a long-term follow-up study, five of ten children older than 11 years of age reported that their dizziness attacks had stopped (Krams et al. 2011). Frequently, there are transitions to other forms of migraine with and without aura (Lanzi et al. 1994; Zhang et al. 2012). Basilar-type migraine also peaks in incidence during adolescence (Bickerstaff 1961). About 50 % of children with dizziness also have headache (Balatsouras et al. 2007). Episodic ataxia type 2 can imitate benign paroxysmal vertigo in childhood (Bertholon et al. 2010).

The therapy of choice for frequent attacks of benign paroxysmal vertigo in childhood is the analogous migraine prophylaxis administered to adults with vestibular migraine, which may lead to a significant improvement (Baier et al. 2009). In our experience, magnesium (2 mg/kg/day) is evidently also effective in children.

6.1.4   Episodic Ataxias

So far, seven forms of episodic ataxias (EA) have been described (Griggs and Nutt 1995; Jen 2008). They are mostly autosomally dominant diseases. The main symptom is recurrent attacks with ataxia in combination with cerebellar and/or vestibular disorders even in the attack-free interval. EA2 is clearly the most frequent form, whereas EA1 is very rare. The other forms have been described to occur in only a few families.

EA1 is characterized by recurring attacks with ataxia and interictal neuro-myokymia (Brunt and van Weerden 1990); it is based on mutations of the potassium channel. The neuro-myokymia and in part even the attacks in EA1 can be successfully treated with potassium channel blockers like phenytoin or carbamazepine. In addition, acetazolamide can be administered in daily doses of 62.5–1,000 mg to avoid attacks (overview in Jen et al. (2007)). The effect of acetazolamide is probably due to an alteration of the pH value, in the sense of an acidosis, that leads, for example, to reduced potassium conductivity.

EA2 is the clinically most relevant subtype and is an important differential diagnosis for vestibular migraine (Sect. 3.2). As a rule, EA2 manifests in late childhood or in early adulthood. The attacks generally last for hours or up to one day. The typical triggers are sports, stress, or alcohol. EA2 is caused by mutations in the so-called PQ calcium channel gene on chromosome 19p13; this is found in only 60–70 % of all clinically confirmed diagnoses (Jen et al. 2004). Attacks are prevented by avoiding physical exertion, emotional stress, and alcohol.

Acetazolamide and 4-aminopyridine are used for prophylaxis. Acetazolamide is effective in 70 % of the cases (dosage 250–1,000 mg/day); however, there are still no controlled studies available (Griggs et al. 1978; Brandt and Strupp 1997; Strupp et al. 2007). The drug's efficacy declines in many patients after 1–2 years, or the treatment has to be stopped due to undesired side effects, especially kidney stones.

In an open application of 4-aminopyridine, it was observed for the first time that the potassium channel blocker had a positive effect on EA2 (Strupp et al. 2004). Later, a placebo-controlled, double-blind, crossover study showed that 4-aminopyridine at a dosage of 3×5 mg/day significantly reduces the number of attacks and improves the life quality (Strupp et al. 2011). The drug's mechanism of action was investigated in animal models: 4-aminopyridine led to a normalization of the irregular discharging of the Purkinje cells in mutant mice (Alvina and Khodakhah 2010). Treatment with this low dosage is tolerated well. It is important before beginning the treatment to perform an EKG after administering a test dose: the QTc time must not be lengthened. The retard form of 4-AP can also be used as an alternative (fampridine, 1–2×10 mg/day). Treatment with the aminopyridines is in each case a nonstandard individual treatment strategy.

6.1.5   Motion Sickness

Children younger than 2 years of age are seldom affected by motion sickness. Later and until puberty, however, they are more susceptible to motion sickness when riding in a vehicle than are adults (see Sect. 6.4).

6.2   Drug-Induced Vertigo

Vertigo is frequently caused by medicine, a possibility that is generally underestimated (Table 6.3). The key to diagnosis of such cases is a carefully taken patient history. The temporal relationship between the onset of the respective drug treatment and the occurrence of symptoms is especially important (if suspected, try drug elimination). The "reverse" method of identifying associations between dizziness and the causative drugs, which Blakley and Gulati (2008) proposed, seems of little help, practically speaking. As the complaints and the clinical picture greatly differ and the underlying mode of action of many drugs that induce vertigo is unclear, there is still no satisfactory classification of drug-induced vertigo:

- On the one hand, certain drugs are known to have ototoxic effects, such as the aminoglycosides, which cause direct (practically selective) damage of the hair cells (see Sect. 2.6).
- On the other hand, drugs such as anticonvulsants (e.g., carbamazepine and diphenylhydantoin) cause pronounced central (dose dependent) ocular motor disorders, although according to their principal mode of action, they affect all neurons of the central nervous system (overview in Rascol et al. 1995; Cianfrone et al. 2011). Clinical neurological investigations frequently show that the latter mostly cause saccadic smooth pursuit and a gaze-holding deficit in all directions (see Sect. 1.7).

Table 6.3 Drug groups that can cause vertigo as a side effect

Nervous and musculoskeletal systems	Heart, blood vessels, blood
Anticonvulsants	Beta-receptor blockers
Analgesics	Antiarrhythmics
Tranquilizers	Vasodilators/vasoconstrictors
Muscle relaxants	Anticoagulants
Hypnotics	**Kidneys and bladder**
Antiemetics	Diuretics
Antidepressants	Spasmolytics
Anticholinergics	**Respiratory organs**
Dopamine agonists	Expectorants
Antiphlogistics	Antitussives
Local anesthetics	Bronchospasm relaxants
Hormones	Mucus dissolvents
Corticosteroids	**Miscellaneous**
Antidiabetics	Antiallergics
Gonadal hormones	Prostaglandins
Oral contraceptives	X-ray contrast media
Inflammations	
Antibiotics	
Tuberculostatics	
Antihelmintics	
Antifungals	

Antihypertensives and diuretics are also relevant, as they can lead to orthostatic dysregulation. Many patients experience this dysregulation as a brief, temporary postural vertigo when they sit up; it can lead to falls (overview in Tinetti 2002). The diagnosis can be supported by the Schellong test. Table 6.3 presents a selection of drug groups that elicit the undesired side effect of vertigo.

Above all, the elderly can have vertigo as a side effect of drugs, for example, a cardiovascular drug or medicine that acts on the central nervous system (Shoair et al. 2011).

6.3 Cervicogenic Vertigo

Somatosensors in the muscles, joints, and skin can also induce sensations of self-motion and trigger nystagmus. Vision satisfactorily substitutes for sensory loss caused by disorders such as polyneuropathy or spinal cord diseases and thus ensures spatial orientation and postural control in the daytime; however, in darkness or under poor visual conditions, disturbed proprioception typically causes postural imbalance, dizziness or vertigo. There is, therefore, also a somatosensory vertigo.

The clinical picture of a cervicogenic vertigo, triggered solely by a disorder of the neck afferents, is still controversial (Sect. 4.3), although the important contribution of these receptors to spatial orientation, postural control, and head–trunk coordination is well known.

The difficulty of clinical evaluation is based on:

- Insufficient pathophysiological knowledge of function and multimodal interaction of the sensory signals from the neck afferents
- The existing conceptual confusion about the so-called cervical vertigo (Brandt 1996; Brandt and Bronstein 2001)

The neural connections between the neck receptors and the central vestibular system—the cervico-ocular reflex and the neck reflexes for postural control—have been investigated experimentally; however, so far, the findings have had little clinical relevance. In humans, unilateral anesthesia of the deep posterolateral neck region (e.g., C2 blocks for cervicogenic headache) causes a transient ataxia accompanied by ipsiversive deviation of gait and past-pointing without spontaneous nystagmus (Dieterich et al. 1993). It is difficult to apply these findings to patients with occipital neck/head pain and postural and gait imbalance, because the diagnosis cannot yet be confirmed. The recommended neck-turning test along with examination of the static cervico-ocular reflex or Romberg's test of stance while the patient leans his head backward is nonspecific and insufficiently standardized (De Jong and Bles 1986). It was shown, for example, that turning the trunk induces nystagmus in patients with a cervical syndrome as often as it does in healthy controls (Holtmann et al. 1993). Optimistic reports that cannot be confirmed by the current literature on the frequency of cervicogenic vertigo and the fantastic successes achieved by chiropractic treatment must be carefully assessed.

The mostly controversial debate about the reality or fiction of cervicogenic vertigo resembles a "war between believers and doubters" lacking any corresponding practical significance. The cervical syndrome is treated by drugs and physical therapy, and once other causes are excluded, the hypothetical neurophysiological explanation mentioned above is still mainly only of theoretical significance.

6.4 Motion Sickness

6.4.1 Clinical Aspects and Pathogenesis

Acute motion sickness arises during passive transportation in vehicles; it resolves spontaneously within 1 day at the most after the disappearance of the inducing stimulus (Fig. 6.1). The full picture of acute severe motion sickness evolves with initial symptoms of:

- Light-headedness
- Physical discomfort
- Tiredness
- Periodic yawning
- Pallor
- Light dizziness with apparent surround motion and self-motion

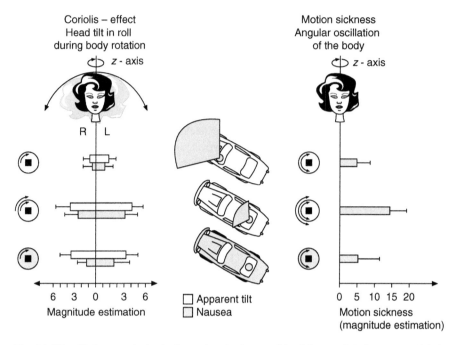

Fig. 6.1 Visual influences during body acceleration in a combined drum and chair system and their effects on vertigo and motion sickness. Magnitude estimations of apparent tilt and nausea induced by sideward tilts of the head during simultaneous body rotation while sitting. Coriolis effects are induced in the process by the cross-coupled accelerations (*left*). Magnitude estimation of motion sickness induced by 15 min of sinusoidal angular oscillation of the body on a rotatory chair with a frequency of 0.02 Hz and peak velocity of 100°/s. The three visual conditions were eyes open (*top*), rotary chair and drum movements mechanically coupled (*middle*), and eyes open in complete darkness (*bottom*). The experimentally induced nausea was greatest when the vestibular and visual information on movement was contradictory (combined movement of chair and drum). This corresponds to the experience in moving vehicles (*right*). Motion sickness is least pronounced when vision can simultaneously check body acceleration (in the driver seat); conversely, motion sickness is greatest when the vestibular acceleration apparently contradicts visual information (in the back seat with predominantly stationary contrasts in the visual field or when reading) (reproduced with permission from Brandt et al. (1976))

An increase in facial pallor is followed by cold sweats, increased salivation, hypersensitivity to smells, occipital head pain, and feelings of pressure in the upper abdomen. Finally, the central symptoms of nausea, retching, and vomiting develop with motor incoordination, loss of drive and concentration, apathy, and fear of impending doom (Money 1970).

Motion sickness is not caused by vestibular "overstimulation" during strong accelerations of the body, but by unfamiliar (i.e., non-adapted) motion stimuli and particularly by intersensory perceptual incongruencies among the visual, vestibular, and somatosensory systems. The most important concept explaining the pathogenesis of motion sickness is the so-called mismatch theory (Reason 1978; Dichgans and Brandt 1978). According to this theory, the decisive trigger is the incongruence of the signals of motion from various sensory channels or the incongruence between expected and actual sensory stimulation.

New experiments suggest that the spatial orientation of the velocity storage of the vestibulo-ocular reflex plays a role in the generation of motion sickness due to head movements (Dai et al. 2007). Well-known varieties of motion sickness are:

- Car sickness (visual–vestibular conflict of stimuli)
- Seasickness (unfamiliar, complex linear, and angular accelerations of low frequency, below 1 Hz)
- Vehicle simulator sickness (optokinetic motion sickness)
- Space sickness (incongruent sensory stimuli of the otoliths, semicircular canals, and the visual system during active head movements in microgravity)

Epidemiological studies have found a statistically significant association of migraine and susceptibility to motion sickness (Neuhauser and Lempert 2004; Evans et al. 2007; Cuomo-Granston and Drummond 2010), above all in vestibular migraine patients (Boldingh et al. 2011).

6.4.2 Course and Therapy

Despite considerable interindividual variation in resistance, every healthy individual can experience motion sickness when exposed to extreme acceleration stimuli (e.g., cross-coupled acceleration like the Coriolis effects). Figures on the incidence of motion sickness in different motor vehicles vary between 1 and 90 %. During the first days of an Atlantic crossing with moderate turbulence, about 25–30 % of ship passengers experience motion sickness, whereas 80 % of subjects on small life rafts or adrift with flotation vests become severely seasick. The latter's survival chances are reduced by the additional loss of water and electrolytes. Women are more susceptible than men, and children and young adults are more susceptible than the aged. Newborns and infants up to the age of 1 year are extremely resistant to motion sickness, apparently because they use the visual system for dynamic space orientation only after they have learned to stand alone and walk. Thus, they do not experience any visual–vestibular conflict of perception while being transported in a vehicle (Brandt 1976). Loss of labyrinthine function causes resistance to motion sickness, whereas blindness does not.

Motion sickness is an acute clinical syndrome. Nausea and vomiting develop within minutes to hours, and the symptoms show spontaneous remission within hours to 1 day after the stimulus ceases. If the stimulus continues (ship or space travel), relief occurs via centrally mediated adaptation (habituation) within 3 days.

The *mal-de-debarquement syndrome* is a stance and gait unsteadiness with postural vertigo that develops on land after longer ship travel (Brown and Baloh 1987; Murphy 1993; Cha 2009). Moeller and Lempert (2007) speculated that it has to do with pseudohallucinations of the "vestibular memory." Such complaints can occur at short notice in the form of sensorimotor aftereffects even in healthy subjects after a long-persisting motion stimulus (e.g., "seamen's legs"). Patients suffering from this condition exhibit impaired postural stability, kinesiophobia, and fatigue (Clark et al. 2013). In FDG PET and fMRI, they show an association between resting-state metabolic activity and functional connectivity between the entorhinal cortex and amygdala (Cha et al. 2012). The syndrome lasts for months or years with a substantial economic burden (Macke et al. 2012) and recalls the development of somatoform vertigo similar to that of phobic postural vertigo. Repetitive transcranial magnetic stimulation has been tried for therapy with some short-term improvement of mal-de-debarquement symptoms (Cha et al. 2013). However, diagnostically the condition can easily be confused with phobic postural vertigo (Sect. 5.2).

The most effective physical means of prevention of motion sickness is adaptation (habituation) by intermittent exposure to the stimulus. This adaptation, however, is only temporary and specific for each type of acceleration, i.e., resistance to seasickness does not protect from flight sickness.

If "vestibular training" (http://extra.springer.com) does not make the subject resistant, his/her head should be kept still during the stimulus, and additional accelerations that are complexly coupled with the vehicle motion should be avoided. Susceptibility is less when lying than when sitting (Golding et al. 1995).

Motion sickness develops above all in closed vehicles or while reading on the back seat of a car, when the body is being accelerated, but a stationary environment is being viewed, which contradicts the labyrinthine stimuli. By maintaining adequate visual control of the vehicle movement, one can significantly reduce motion sickness from that experienced under eyes-closed conditions. Conversely, susceptibility is significantly increased if primarily stationary contrasts fill the field of vision (Dichgans and Brandt 1973; Probst et al. 1982).

Antivertiginous drugs such as dimenhydrinate (Dramamine) or scopolamine (Transderm Scop) can inhibit the spontaneous activity of the neurons of the vestibular nuclei as well as the neuronal frequency modulation during body acceleration, thus reducing the susceptibility to motion sickness.

6.4.3   Pragmatic Therapy

The possibilities of physical prevention and pharmacological measures (Bles et al. 2000; Shupak and Gordon 2006; Spinks and Wasiak 2011; Huppert et al. 2011; Murdin et al. 2011) are listed in Tables 6.4 and 6.5. As a transdermal therapeutic system (TTS), scopolamine is the preferred drug for prophylaxis. If applied in patch form, it must be stuck to the skin (e.g., behind the ear) 4–8 h before traveling because of the delayed release of the active agent. Scopolamine is more effective than cinnarizine (Gil et al. 2012) or dimenhydrinate. Doubling the usual single doses (100 mg dimenhydrinate, 0.6 mg scopolamine) clearly increases the central sedating side effects without causing any essential improvement in resistance to motion sickness (Wood et al. 1966). The effect of the individual substances can be intensified in severe cases by combining an antihistamine with a sympathicomimetic drug

Table 6.4 Physical maneuvers to prevent motion sickness

Measure	Goal
Before	
"Vestibular training" by repeated exposure to stimulus and active head movements	Movement-specific central habituation
Vehicle simulator training	Utilization of the visual–vestibular transfer of habituation
Acute	
Fixation of the head	Avoidance of additional accelerations, which are complexly coupled with vehicle acceleration (e.g., Coriolis effect)
Head position (toward the vector of gravitation) Ship: supine Car: supine with head in direction of movement Helicopter: sitting position	Utilization of the head-axis specific difference in resistance to the acceleration, acceleration along the z-axis most favorable
Possible counter-regulation of the body motion induced by vehicle acceleration (e.g., inclining toward the curve)	
Visual control of the vehicle movement; if not possible, then close the eyes	Avoidance of a visual–vestibular conflict (mismatch) of perception

Table 6.5 Drug prophylaxis for motion sickness

Drugs	Side effects
Antihistamine 100 mg dimenhydrinate (Dramamine)	Sedation, reduced reactions and concentration, dryness of the mouth, blurred vision, light-headedness
Belladonna alkaloids 0.5 mg scopolamine as transdermal therapeutic system (Transderm Scop) 4–6 h before trip onset effective up to 72 h	

(25 mg promethazine and 25 mg amphetamine) (Wood and Graybiel 1970). Phenytoin was also tested for efficacy against motion sickness (Knox et al. 1994); however, in view of its side effects, it is not recommended (Murdin et al. 2011).

6.5 Height Vertigo and Acrophobia

6.5.1 Clinical Aspects and Pathogenesis

Physiological height vertigo is a visually induced destabilization of stance and locomotion accompanied by individually various amounts of strong anxiety and vegetative symptoms at the sight of towers, ladders, buildings, a cliff, or a mountain ridge. In Anglo-American countries, height vertigo ("fear of heights" or "acrophobia") is classified as a variant of specific phobias in accordance with the criteria of the "Diagnostic and Statistical Manual of Mental Disorders" (DSM IV). In a large prospective study, the lifetime prevalence for acrophobia was reported to lie between 3.1 and 5.3 % (Curtis et al. 1998; Depla et al. 2008). However, there is certainly a continuum stretching from acrophobia to a less pronounced but stimulus-dependent visual height intolerance that does not fulfill the diagnostic criteria of a specific phobia (Salassa and Zapala 2009; Coelho and Wallis 2010; Brandt et al. 2012b).

The prevalence of this individual susceptibility was determined for the first time in a population-relevant survey of more than 3,000 persons (Huppert et al. 2013). The important findings were as follows:

- The prevalence of visual height intolerance in the general population amounts to 28 % (women 32 %, men 25 %).
- Height intolerance appears most frequently in the second decade (30 %); the first manifestation can, however, occur throughout the entire life span.
- Climbing up a tower is the most frequent initial stimulus, followed by climbing ladders, mountain hiking, or looking from high buildings. With time, there is an increase in the spectrum of the stimuli in more than 50 %.
- More than 50 % of those affected develop an avoidance behavior of certain stimuli, i.e., they limit their physical activities.
- Only 11 % consult a physician for their complaints.
- The prevalence of migraine amounts to 21 % in persons with height intolerance, whereas in the general population, it occurs in 12–14 %.

Although height vertigo has so far been considered mainly a phobia, there is a physiological explanation for the postural instability and vertigo caused by optical stimuli at the sight of free-standing buildings (Fig. 6.2) (Bles et al. 1980; Brandt et al. 1980). Physiological visual height imbalance is rather a "distance vertigo" caused by "visual destabilization" of upright posture, when the distance between the observer's eyes and the nearest visible stationary contrasts within the field of vision becomes critically large. Then head and body sway can no longer be corrected by vision, since the movements cannot be registered by the sensors due to the subthreshold smallness of the retinal shift. The vestibular and somatosensory signals of a shifting of the body's center of gravity over the standing surface contradict the visual information of preserved body stability. Under such stimulus conditions, the body sway is measurably increased, and above all, the visual postural reflexes to the disturbing input are so impaired that there is real danger of an accident or fall. The critical stimulus parameters of the trigger and also practical pointers for prophylaxis can be derived from this physiological mechanism (Table 6.5). The following three terms could be used to distinguish different states of physiological and psychopathological mechanisms active during exposure to heights (Brandt et al. 2012a):

- Physiological visual height imbalance of posture which concerns everyone
- Visual height intolerance, which occurs in one of three and is more or less distressing
- Acrophobia or fear of heights, defined as a specific phobia, which affects four in 100 and represents the severest end of the spectrum of visual height intolerance

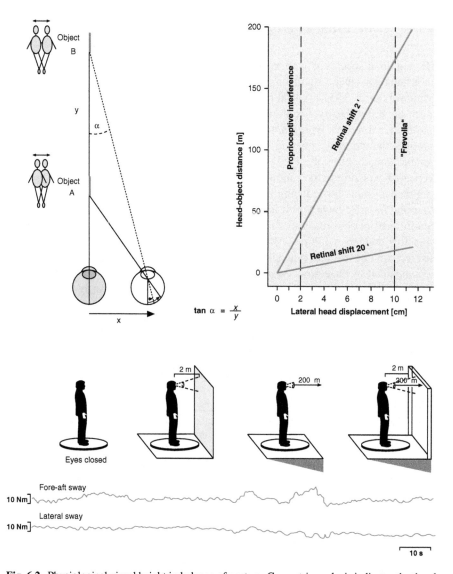

Fig. 6.2 Physiological visual height imbalance of posture. Geometric analysis indicates that head sway with respect to the surroundings is visually detected with more difficulty if the distance between eyes and surrounding contrasts increases. When objects are fixated, the same geometric relationship pertains for efferent and also reafferent perception of the eye movements triggered by the head sway. Actually there is a reinforcement of the posturographically measurable body sway under such visual conditions (*below*). Fore–aft and lateral body sway is minimal with eyes open 2 m in front of a structured wall and maximal when looking into the distance without nearby contrasts. As soon as nearby stationary contrasts appear in the visual field periphery while gazing in the distance, they are used for the visual stabilization of stance (reproduced with permission from Brandt et al. (1980))

6.5.2 Course and Therapy

Many animal species as well as humans have a largely gene-based fear and avoidance behavior when visually approaching a step or an abyss (visual-cliff phenomenon; Walk et al. 1957). Visual height intolerance is accordingly physiological and must be differentiated from pathological acrophobia. Subjective visual height intolerance develops within a matter of only seconds after a glance into an abyss, but once the inducing situation disappears, it rapidly resolves. The latter phenomenon has already been observed in Chinese and Greek Antiquity (Bauer et al. 2012). Repeated exposure to the stimulus can lead to a certain amount of adaptation.

Practical hints for reducing physiological height vertigo are given in Table 6.6. Acrophobia arises when physiological height imbalance or intolerance induces a conditioned phobic reaction characterized by a dissociation of the subjective and objective danger of falling. Although the acrophobic patient also recognizes this discrepancy, he/she can typically only with difficulty overcome the panic anxiety accompanied by vegetative symptoms and inappropriate avoidance behavior. Drugs such as tranquilizers or antidepressants can only be used temporarily as support.

Psychotherapy for acrophobia and also agoraphobia is dominated by behavioral therapy approaches, which can be classified as either systematic or in vivo desensibilization strategies (Table 6.7); "virtual reality" exposure is also used (Pull 2005). The method of systematic desensibilization (Wolpe 1958) is based on the creation of a

Table 6.6 Visual height imbalance of posture and height intolerance ("height vertigo")

Mechanism	Distance vertigo with visual destabilization of body balance if the distance between eyes and the nearest stationary objects exceeds 3 m (if physiological height imbalance induces a conditioned phobic reaction, then acrophobia (fear of heights) develops)
Features	
Body posture	Strongest when standing without support, weakest when lying, increases during extreme tilts of the head
Height	Begins after ca. 3 m, maximal more than ca. 20 m
Gradient	Begins after 40–50°, maximal after 70–80° slope of the ground
Gaze direction	Postural instability also occurs when gazing upward; decisive is the distance between eyes and object
Prevention	
Body posture	Improvement of posture stabilization by leaning on something, holding tight to something, or sitting down, particularly if there are additional disturbing stimuli such as wind; avoid extreme inclinations of the head in order to keep the otoliths in optimal operating position
Vision	Look at near stationary contrasts; when looking into the abyss, keep near stationary objects in sight in the peripheral field of vision in order to maintain visual control of posture; avoid large-field motion stimuli (clouds) that can lead to visually induced illusory motion; when in danger of falling, do not look through binoculars without some kind of support/stabilization

Table 6.7 Behavioral therapy for acrophobia

Systematic desensitization	Presentation of graduated hierarchy of imagined anxiety-provoking visual scenes during muscle relaxation, which has been trained earlier
In vivo desensitization	
Successive approximation	Gradual approach to situations provoking anxiety with the help of instructions and reinforcement under conditions close to reality
Contact desensitization	The therapist subjects himself while in close physical contact with the patient to the same provoking situation and serves as a model
Flooding	Direct confrontation of the patient with the strongest provoking situations under real-life conditions as long as possible

graduated hierarchy of visual scenes that cause anxiety. These scenes are then presented to the patients during a period of calm after they have "absolved a training phase of muscle relaxation." In vivo desensibilization procedures, in which anxiety is supposed to be reduced during provoking situations that are close to life and not imagined, are, however, more effective. The stepwise approach ("successive approximation") to the fear-inducing situation is supported by instructions and reinforcement. The so-called contact desensibilization (Ritter 1969) especially stresses the advantages of the therapist's participation and physical nearness, which serves as a model for the patient ("participant modeling") during the graduated approach to situations triggering height vertigo. An alternative method is the patient's in vivo confrontation with the strongest provoking situation for as long as possible, so-called flooding. There are first indications that the glucocorticoids can improve psychotherapy for "fear removal" in cases of acrophobia (de Quervain et al. 2011). Cumulative histories of patients with phobias which showed that even without psychotherapy most childhood phobias and also 40–60 % of adult phobias improve spontaneously or resolve after an interval of 5–6 years (Agras et al. 1972; Noyes et al. 1980) may be too optimistic.

References

Abu-Arafeh I, Russel G. Paroxysmal vertigo as a migraine equivalent in children: a population-based study. Cephalalgia. 1995;15:22–5.

Agras WS, Chapin HN, Oliveau DC. The natural history of phobia. Arch Gen Psychiatry. 1972;26:315–7.

Alvina K, Khodakhah K. The therapeutic mode of action of 4-aminopyridine in cerebellar ataxia. J Neurosci. 2010;30:7258–68.

American Psychiatric Association. Diagnostic and statistical manual of mental disorders (DSM IV). 4th ed. Washington: American Psychiatric Association; 1994.

Baier B, Winkenwerder E, Dieterich M. Vestibular migraine: effects of prophylactic therapy with various drugs. A retrospective study. J Neurol. 2009;256:426–42.

Balatsouras DG, Kaberos A, Assimakopoulos D, Katotomichelakis M, Economou NC, Korres SG. Etiology of vertigo in children. Int J Pediatr Otorhinolaryngol. 2007;71:487–94.

Basser LS. Benign paroxysmal vertigo of childhood. A variety of vestibular neuronitis. Brain. 1964;87:141–52.

Bauer M, Huppert D, Brandt T. Fear of heights in ancient China. J Neurol. 2012;259:2223–5.

Bertholon P, Chabrier S, Riant F, Tournier-Lasserve E, Peyron R. Episodic ataxia type 2: unusual aspects in clinical and genetic presentation. Special emphasis in childhood. J Neurol Neurosurg Psychiatry. 2010;80:1289–92.

Bickerstaff ER. Basilar artery migraine. Lancet. 1961;1:15–8.

Blakley BW, Gulati H. Identifying drugs that cause dizziness. Otolaryngology. 2008;37:11–5.

Bles W, Kapteyn TS, Brandt T, Arnold F. The mechanism of physiological height vertigo: II. Posturography. Acta Otolaryngol (Stockh). 1980;89:534–40.

Bles W, Bos JE, Kruit H. Motion sickness. Curr Opin Neurol. 2000;13:19–25.

Boldingh MI, Ljostad U, Mygland A, Monstad P. Vestibular sensitivity in vestibular migraine: VEMP's and motion sickness susceptibility. Cephalalgia. 2011;31:1211–9.

Brandt T. Optisch-vestibuläre Bewegungskrankheit, Höhenschwindel und klinische Schwindelformen. Fortschr Med. 1976;94:177–1188.

Brandt T. Cervical vertigo – reality or fiction? Audiol Neurotol. 1996;1:187–96.

Brandt T, Bronstein AM. Cervical vertigo. J Neurol Neurosurg Psychiatry. 2001;71:8–12.

Brandt T, Strupp M. Episodic ataxia type 1 and 2 (familial periodic ataxia/vertigo). Audiol Neurotol. 1997;2:373–83.

Brandt T, Wenzel D, Dichgans J. Die Entwicklung der visuellen Stabilisation des aufrechten Standes beim Kind: Ein Reifezeichen in der Kinderneurologie. Arch Psychiat Nervenkr. 1976;223:1–13.

Brandt T, Arnold F, Bles W, Kapteyn TS. The mechanism of physiological height vertigo: I.Theoretical approach and psychophysics. Acta Otolaryngol (Stockh). 1980;89:513–23.

Brandt T, Benson J, Huppert D. What to call "non-phobic" fear of heights? Br J Psychiatry. 2012a;190:81. doi:10.1192/bjp190.1.81a.

Brandt T, Strupp M, Huppert D. Height intolerance – an underrated threat. J Neurol. 2012b;259: 759–60.

Brown JJ, Baloh RW. Persistent mal de debarquement-syndrome: a motion-induced subjective disorder of balance. Am J Otolaryngol. 1987;8:219–22.

Brunt ER, van Weerden TW. Familial paroxysmal kinesiogenic ataxia and continuous myokymia. Brain. 1990;113:1361–82.

Cha YH. Mal de debarquement. Semin Neurol. 2009;29:520–7.

Cha YH, Chakrapani S, Craig A, Baloh RW. Metabolic and functional connectivity changes in mal de debarquement syndrome. PLoS One. 2012;7:e49560.

Cha YH, Cui Y, Baloh RW. Repetitive transcranial magnetic stimulation for mal de debarquement syndrome. Otol Neurotol. 2013;34:175–9.

Cianfrone G, Pentangelo D, Cianfrone E, Mazzei F, Turchetta R, Orlando MP, et al. Pharmacological drugs inducing ototoxicity, vestibular symptoms and tinnitus: a reasoned and update guide. Eur Rev Med Pharmacol Sci. 2011;15:601–36.

Clark BC, Leporte A, Clark S, Hoffman RL, Quick A, Wilson TE, et al. Effects of persistent mal de debarquement syndrome on balance, psychological traits, and motor cortex excitability. J Clin Neurosci. 2013;20:446–50.

Coelho CM, Wallis G. Deconstructing acrophobia: physiological and psychological precursors to developing a fear of heights. Depress Anxiety. 2010;27:864–70.

Cuomo-Granston A, Drummond PD. Migraine and motion sickness: what is the link? Prog Neurobiol. 2010;91:300–12.

Curtis GC, Magee WJ, Eaton WW, Wittchen HU. Specific fears and phobias. Epidemiology and classification. Br J Psychiatry. 1998;173:212–7.

Dai M, Raphan T, Cohen B. Labyrinthine lesions and motion sickness susceptibility. Exp Brain Res. 2007;178:477–87.

De Jong IMBV, Bles W. Cervical dizziness and ataxia. In: Bles W, Brandt T, editors. Disorders of posture and gait. Amsterdam/New York/Oxford: Elsevier; 1986. p. 185–206.

De Quervain DJ, Bentz D, Michael T, Bolt OC, Wiederhold BK, Margraf J, et al. Glucocorticoids enhance extinction-based psychotherapy. Proc Natl Acad Sci. 2011;108:6621–5.

Depla MFIA, ten Have ML, van Balkom AJLM, de Graf R. Specific fears and phobias in the general population: results from the Netherlands Mental Health Survey and Incidence Study (NEMESIS). Soc Psychiatry Psychiatr Epidemiol. 2008;43:200–8.

Dichgans J, Brandt T. Optokinetic motion-sickness and pseudo-coriolis effects induced by moving visual stimuli. Acta Otolaryngol. 1973;76:339–48.

Dichgans J, Brandt T. Visual-vestibular interaction: effects of self-motion perception and postural control. In: Held R, Leibowitz HW, Teuber HL, editors. Handbook of Sensory Physiology, Perception, vol. III. Berlin/Heidelberg/New York: Springer; 1978. p. 755–804.

Dieterich M, Pöllmann W, Pfaffenrath V. Cervicogenic headache: electronystagmography, perception of verticality and posturography in patients before and after C2-blockade. Cephalalgia. 1993;13:285–8.

Erbek SH, Erbek SS, Yilmaz I, Topal O, Ozgirgin N, Ozluoglu LN, et al. Vertigo in childhood: a clinical experience. Int J Pediatr Otorhinolaryngol. 2006;70:1547–54.

Evans RW, Marcus D, Furman JM. Motion sickness and migraine. Headache. 2007;47: 607–10.

Gil A, Nachum Z, Tal D, Shupak A. A comparison of cinnarizine and transdermal scopolamine for the prevention of seasickness in a naval crew: a double-blind, randomized, crossover study. Clin Neuropharmacol. 2012;35:37–9.

Golding IF, Markey HM, Stott IR. The effects of motion direction, body axis, and posture on motion sickness induced by low frequency linear oscillation. Aviat Space Environ Med. 1995;66:1046–51.

Griggs RC, Nutt JG. Episodic ataxias as channelopathies. Ann Neurol. 1995;37:285–7.

Griggs RC, Moxley RT, Lafrance RA, McQuillen J. Hereditary paroxysmal ataxia: response to acetazolamide. Neurology. 1978;28:1259–64.

Holtmann S, Reiman V, Schöps P. Clinical significance of cervico-ocular reactions. Laryngorhinootologie. 1993;72:306–10.

Huppert D, Strupp M, Mückter H, Brandt T. Which medication do I need to manage dizzy patients? Acta Otolaryngol. 2011;131:228–41.

Huppert D, Grill E, Brandt T. Down on heights? One in three has visual height intolerance. J Neurol. 2013;260:597–604.

Jahn K, Zwergal A, Strupp M, Brandt T. Schwindel im Kindesalter. Nervenheilkunde. 2009;28:47–52.

Jahn K, Langhagen T, Schroeder AS, Heinen F. Vertigo and dizziness in childhood – update on diagnosis and treatment. Neuropediatrics. 2011;42:129–34.

Jen JC. Hereditary episodic ataxias. Ann N Y Acad Sci. 2008;1142:250–3.

Jen J, Kim GW, Baloh RW. Clinical spectrum of episodic ataxia type 2. Neurology. 2004;62:17–22.

Jen JC, Graves TD, Hess EJ, Hanna MG, Griggs RC, Baloh RW. Primary episodic ataxias: diagnosis, pathogenesis and treatment. Brain. 2007;130:2484–93.

Kanaan AA, Raad RA, Hourani RG, Zaytoun GM. Bilateral superior semicircular canal dehiscence in a child with sensorineural hearing loss and without vestibular symptoms. Int J Pediatr Otorhinolaryngol. 2011;75:877–9.

Knox GW, Woodard D, Chelen W, Ferguson R, Johnson L. Phenytoin for motion sickness: clinical evaluation. Laryngoscope. 1994;1994:935–9.

Krams B, Echenne B, Leydet J, Rivier F, Roubertie A. Benign paroxysmal vertigo of childhood: long-term outcome. Cephalalgia. 2011;31:439–43.

Lanzi G, Balottin U, Fazzi E, Tagliasacchi M, Manfrin M, Mira E. Benign paroxysmal vertigo of childhood: a long-term follow-up. Cephalalgia. 1994;14:458–60.

Lee GS, Zhou G, Poe D, Kenna M, Amin M, Ohlms L, et al. Clinical experience in diagnosis and management of superior semicircular canal dehiscence in children. Laryngoscope. 2011;121:2256–61.

Macke A, LePorte A, Clark BC. Social, societal, and economic burden of mal de debarquement syndrome. J Neurol. 2012;259:1326–30.

Moeller L, Lempert T. Mal de debarquement: pseudo-hallucinations from vestibular memory? J Neurol. 2007;254:813–5.

Money KE. Motion sickness. Physiol Rev. 1970;50:1–39.

Murdin L, Golding J, Bronstein A. Managing motion sickness. BMJ. 2011;343:d7430.

Murphy TP. Mal de debarquement syndrome: a forgotten entity? Otolaryngol Head Neck Surg. 1993;109:10–3.

Neuhauser H, Lempert T. Vertigo and dizziness related to migraine: a diagnostic challenge. Cephalalgia. 2004;24:83–91.

Niemensivu R, Kentala E, Wiener-Vacher S, Pyykko I. Evaluation of vertiginous children. Eur Arch Otorhinolaryngol. 2007;264:1129–35.

Noyes R, Clancy J, Hoenk PR, Slymen DJ. The prognosis of anxiety neurosis. Arch Gen Psychiatry. 1980;37:173–8.

Probst T, Krafczyk S, Büchele W, Brandt T. Visuelle Prävention der Bewegungskrankheit im Auto. Arch Psychiat Nervenkr. 1982;231:409–21.

Pull CB. Current status of virtual reality exposure therapy in anxiety disorders: editorial review. Curr Opin Psychiatry. 2005;18:7–14.

Rascol O, Hain TC, Brefel C, Benazet M, Clanet M, Montastruc JL. Antivertigo medications and drug-induced vertigo. A pharmacological review. Drugs. 1995;50:777–91.

Reason JT. Motion sickness adaptation: a neural mismatch model. J R Soc Med. 1978;71:819–29.

Riina N, Ilmari P, Kentala E. Vertigo and imbalance in children: a retrospective study in a Helsinki University otorhinolaryngology clinic. Arch Otolaryngol Head Neck Surg. 2005;131:996–1000.

Ritter B. Treatment of acrophobia with contact desensibilisation. Behav Res Ther. 1969;7:41–5.

Russel G, Abu-Arafeh I. Paroxysmal vertigo in children- an epidemiological study. Int J Pediatr Otorhinolaryngol. 1999;49(1):105–7.

Salassa JR, Zapala DA. Love and fear of heights: the pathophysiology and psychology of height imbalance. Wilderness Environ Med. 2009;20:378–82.

Shoair OA, Nyandege AN, Slattum PW. Medication-related dizziness in the oder adult. Otolaryngol Clin North Am. 2011;44:455–71.

Shupak A, Gordon CR. Motion sickness: advances in pathogenesis, prediction, prevention, and treatment. Aviat Space Environ Med. 2006;77:1213–23.

Spinks AB, Wasiak J. Scopolamine (hyoscine) for preventing and treating motion sickness. Cochrane Database Syst Rev. 2011;6:CD002851.

Strupp M, Kalla R, Dichgans M, Freilinger T, Glasauer S, Brandt T. Treatment of episodic ataxia type 2 with the potassium channel blocker 4-aminopyridine. Neurology. 2004;62:1623–5.

Strupp M, Zwergal A, Brandt T. Episodic ataxia type 2. Neurotherapeutics. 2007;4:267–73.

Strupp M, Kalla R, Claassen J, Adrion C, Mansmann U, Klopstock T, et al. A randomized trial of 4-aminopyridine in EA2 and related familial episodic ataxias. Neurology. 2011;77:269–75.

Tinetti ME. Preventing falls in elderly persons. N Engl J Med. 2002;348:42–9.

Walk RD, Gibson EJ, Tighe TJ. Behaviour of light- and dark-raised rats on a visual cliff. Science. 1957;126:80–1.

Wolpe J. Psychotherapy by reciprocal inhibition. Stanford: Stanford University Press; 1958.

Wood CD, Graybiel A. Evaluation of antimotion sickness drugs: a new effective remedy revealed. Aerosp Med. 1970;41:932–3.

Wood CD, Graybiel A, Kennedy RS. Comparison of effectiveness of some antimotion sickness drugs using recommended and larger than recommended doses as tested in the slow rotation room. Aerospace Med. 1966;37:259–62.

Zhang D, Fan Z, Han Y, Wang M, Xu L, Luo J, et al. Benign paroxysmal vertigo of childhood: diagnostic value of vestibular test and high stimulus rate auditory brainstem response test. Int J Pediatr Otorhinolaryngol. 2012;76:107–10.

Index

T. Brandt et al., *Vertigo and Dizziness*,
DOI 10.1007/978-0-85729-591-0, © Springer-Verlag London 2013

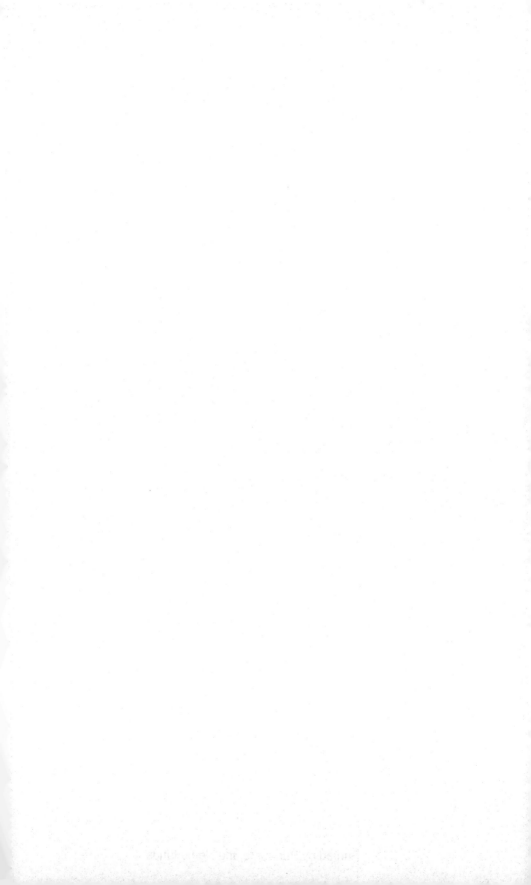

Printed by Printforce, the Netherlands